MILADY STANDARD COSMETOLOGY

Theory
Workbook

MILADY STANDARD COSMETOLOGY

Theory Workbook

To be used with
Milady Standard Cosmetology

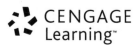
CENGAGE
Learning™

Australia • Brazil • Japan • Korea • Mexico • Singapore • Spain • United Kingdom • United States

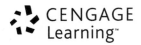
CENGAGE
Learning™

**Milady Standard Cosmetology
Theory Workbook**

President, Milady: Dawn Gerrain

Associate Acquisitions Editor: Philip Mandl

Editorial Assistant: Maria K. Hebert

Director of Beauty Industry Relations:
Sandra Bruce

Executive Marketing Manager: Gerard McAvey

Production Director: Wendy Troeger

Senior Content Project Manager: Angela
Sheehan

Art Director: Benj Gleeksman

Cover Image: © Adrianna Williams/Corbis

For product information and technology assistance, contact us at
Professional & Career Group Customer Support, 1-800-648-7450

For permission to use material from this text or product,
submit all requests online at **www.cengage.com/permissions**
Further permissions questions can be emailed to
permissionrequest@cengage.com

Library of Congress Control Number: 2010903896

ISBN-13: 978-1-4390-5923-4

ISBN-10: 1-4390-5923-3

Milady
5 Maxwell Drive
Clifton Park, NY 12065-2919
USA

Cengage Learning products are represented in Canada by Nelson Education, Ltd.

For your course and learning solutions, visit **milady.cengage.com**

Visit our corporate Web site at **cengage.com.**

Notice to the Reader
Publisher does not warrant or guarantee any of the products described
herein or perform any independent analysis in connection with any of the
product information contained herein. Publisher does not assume, and
expressly disclaims, any obligation to obtain and include information other
than that provided to it by the manufacturer. The reader is expressly warned
to consider and adopt all safety precautions that might be indicated by the
activities described herein and to avoid all potential hazards. By following
the instructions contained herein, the reader willingly assumes all risks in
connection with such instructions. The publisher makes no representations or
warranties of any kind, including but not limited to, the warranties of fitness
for particular purpose or merchantability, nor are any such representations
implied with respect to the material set forth herein, and the publisher takes
no responsibility with respect to such material. The publisher shall not be liable
for any special, consequential, or exemplary damages resulting, in whole or
part, from the readers' use of, or reliance upon, this material.

Printed in the United States of America
6 7 15 14

Contents

How to Use this Workbook

Milady Standard Cosmetology Theory Workbook has been written to meet the needs, interests, and abilities of students receiving training in cosmetology.

This workbook should be used together with *Milady Standard Cosmetology* and *Milady Standard Cosmetology Practical Workbook.* This book directly follows the theoretical information found in the student textbook. Pages to be read and studied are listed at the beginning of each chapter. The practical information can be found in *Milady Standard Cosmetology Practical Workbook.*

Students are to answer each item in this workbook with a pencil after consulting their textbook for correct information. Items can be corrected and/or rated during class or individual discussions, or on an independent study basis.

Various tests are included to emphasize essential facts found in the textbook and to measure the student's progress.

CHAPTER 1 History and Career Opportunities

Date: _____

Rating: _____

Text Pages: 1–15

POINT TO PONDER:

"Remember, determination and enthusiasm triumph over talent and laziness every time."—**Life's Little Instruction Calendar**

WHY STUDY COSMETOLOGY HISTORY AND CAREER OPPORTUNITIES?

1. In your own words, describe why you think it is important for you to learn about old and ancient techniques that were once used in cosmetology.

   _____

   _____

   _____

   _____

   _____

   _____

2. Cosmetologists who know something about the history of their profession are better able to _____ its future.

BRIEF HISTORY OF COSMETOLOGY

3. The term used to encompass a broad range of specialty areas, including hairstyling, nail technology, and esthetics is _____.

4. Define cosmetology. _____

   _____

5. What Greek word is the term *cosmetology* derived from? _____
   What does this term mean? _____

6. Archaeological studies reveal that haircutting and hairstyling were practiced in some form as early as the _____.

7. What ordinary items were used as implements and hair adornment during this time? _____

8. What natural products did ancient people use for coloring matter and tattooing?

_____

9. Who was the first civilized culture to cultivate beauty into an extravagant fashion? _____ For what purposes did they use cosmetics?

_____

_____

10. When was the first evidence of cosmetics in Egypt recorded? _____

a) 3000 BC

b) 2000 BC

c) 1500 BC

d) 1000 BC

11. _____ was an ancient queen who used custom-blended essential oils as her "signature" scents.

12. Which Egyptian queen had a personal cosmetics factory? _____

13. Men in ancient times sometimes stained their nails and lips.

_____ True

_____ False

14. What did Chinese aristocrats rub onto their nails to turn them crimson or ebony?

_____

15. During the Chou Dynasty, what might have happened to people who were not of noble birth if they were caught tinting their nails? _____

_____

16. In 500 BC during the Golden Age of _____, hairstyling became a highly developed art.

17. Greek women applied preparations of _____ on their faces, _____ on their eyes, and _____ on their cheeks and lips.

18. How did the Greeks create the brilliant red pigment named vermillion?

_____

19. In Rome, women used hair color to indicate their class in society. Match the correct shade with its corresponding class:

_____ 1) Noblewomen   a) Black

_____ 2) Middle-class women   b) Red

_____ 3) Poor women   c) Blond

20. During the Middle Ages, where did women not wear colored makeup?

_____ a) Lips

_____ b) Cheeks

_____ c) Eyes

21. Which of the following techniques was originally developed by a physician during the Middle Ages?

_____ a) Croquignole wrapping technique

_____ b) Steam distillation

_____ c) Henna-based hair dyes

_____ d) Cold waving

22. What was discouraged during the Renaissance? _____

_____

23. During the Renaissance, women shaved their eyebrows and hairlines to appear

_____ .

24. During the Victorian Age, what did women use to preserve the health and beauty of the skin? _____ What were they made from?

_____

25. What did Victorian women do to induce natural color rather than use cosmetics?

_____

26. Up until the nineteenth century, barbers performed which of the following services?

_____ a) Minor surgery

_____ b) Haircutting

_____ c) Dentistry

_____ d) All of these answers are correct.

27. Explain the symbolic meaning of the barber pole. _____

_____

_____

_____

_____

_____

28. Up until the end of the nineteenth century, it was common practice for people of both genders to wear wigs.

_____ True

_____ False

29. A _____ would be considered a modern example of a wig.

30. List two major developments that occurred in the early twentieth century that changed Americans' ideas about beauty. 1) _____
2) _____

31. Why was Max Factor's makeup popular with movie stars? _____

_____

32. _____ invented a heavily wired machine that supplied electrical current to metal rods around which hair strands were wrapped.

33. Which of the following methods was most appropriate for use on long hair?

_____ Croquignole wrapping

_____ Spiral wrapping

34. Sarah Breedlove is known for which of the following achievements?

_____ a) Organizing one of the first national meetings for businesswomen in the United States

_____ b) Pioneering the modern African-American hair care and cosmetics industry

_____ c) Devising sophisticated sales and marketing strategies for her hair care products

_____ d) All of these answers are correct.

35. Who invented the curling iron? _____

36. _____ advertisements were initially considered _____ by many women's magazines in the early 1920s.

37. Charles Revson borrowed formulas from what industry to develop his nail polish? _____

38. Name two movie stars who helped make nail polish popular in the 1930s.

_____

39. When was the first permanent haircolor product introduced?

_____ a) 1927

_____ b) 1932

_____ c) 1941

_____ d) 1944

40. Today's alkaline perms are modern versions of what method of permanent waving developed in 1941? _____

41. A term used today that refers to the variety of permanent waving and straightening options for clients is called _____ services.

42. During the 1950s, many women made _____ a regular part of their weekly schedules.

43. This stylist shook the beauty world in the 1960s with his geometric cuts.

_____

44. Which of the following best describes the use of beauty products during the 1980s?

_____ a) Barely there

_____ b) Heavy on the eyeshadow and blush

_____ c) Gentle haircolors in many shades

_____ d) None of these answers are correct.

45. The twenty-first century is currently considered the age of _____ in the beauty industry.

46. Since the late 1980s, the salon industry has evolved to include _____, a term first coined by _____.

47. By 2005, it was commonplace for many salons to use _____ appointment scheduling.

48. Today, most salons use _____ to provide information about their services, location, business hours, and so on to clients and potential clients.

CAREER PATHS FOR COSMETOLOGISTS

49. In addition to attending school, a cosmetologist must be _____ to work as a professional.

50. List eight different areas you may specialize in within the professional industry.

1) _____

2) _____

3) _____

4) _____

5) _____

6) _____

7) _____

8) _____

51. It is a good idea for a specialist to _____ with other reputable _____ as a way of perfecting his or her technique.

52. A salon relies heavily on _____ as a way of staying up-to-date on new trends or techniques within the industry.

53. Having a strong public speaking ability is important for this beauty professional.
_____

54. Explain which of the specialized areas you are most interested in and why.

_____

_____

_____

_____

_____

_____

_____

55. Depending on the specialty area you choose, you may need to join a _____.

56. Describe the skills required of a salon manager. _____

_____

_____

_____

_____

_____

57. The current trend in the cosmetology industry shows a continued _____ in opportunities for professionals.

58. The salon business typically _____ recessions better than other industries.

59. List ways you can make each day in school have a positive impact on your future.

_____

_____

_____

_____

60. Your license will unlock countless doors, but what two things will fuel your career? _____

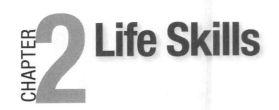

Date: _____

Rating: _____

Text Pages: 16–35

POINT TO PONDER:

"Show up!" Woody Allen said, "90 percent of life is "showing up." Go to class—even when you don't feel like it, when the subject matter seems boring, when you have to bum a ride or take the bus because your car died, when you have a bad hair day or a hangover. Go to class!"

1. The salon is a creative workplace where you will exercise your artistic talent, and it is a highly social atmosphere that will require _____ and excellent _____ .

WHY STUDY LIFE SKILLS?

2. Practicing life skills will lead to a more _____ and _____ career in the beauty industry.

3. Describe in your own words why you think having good life skills will help build your self-esteem.

_____

_____

_____

LIFE SKILLS

4. Below is a list of different life skills. Put a check mark next to the skills you feel you are well on your way to mastering, and put a circle next to the ones you need to improve.

_____

_____

_____

_____

_____ Being genuinely caring and helpful to others

_____ Successfully adapting to different situations

_____ Sticking to a goal and seeing a job to completion

_____ Being consistent with your work

_____ Developing a deep reservoir of common sense

_____ Making good friends

_____ Feeling good about yourself

_____ Maintaining a cooperative attitude

_____ Defining your own code of ethics and living within your definition

_____ Approaching all your work with a strong sense of responsibility

_____ Mastering techniques that will help you become more organized

_____ Having a sense of humor to bring you through difficult situations

_____ Acquiring patience, one of the greatest virtues

_____ Always striving for excellence

5. A "life skill" is a skill you should practice both at work and in your personal life.

_____ True

_____ False

THE PSYCHOLOGY OF SUCCESS

6. All the talent in the world will not make you successful. Talent must be fueled by _____ in order to sustain your career.

7. List the 10 basic principles that form the foundation of all personal and business success.

a) _____

b) _____

c) _____

d) _____

e) _____

f) _____

g) _____

h) _____

i) _____

j) _____

8. How is self-esteem related to success? _____

_____

9. What will help you turn the possibilities in your life into realities? _____

_____

10. How can you maintain a positive self-image? _____

_____

11. You should not depend on how other people define success. How do you define success?

_____

_____

_____

_____

12. How can you develop success? _____

_____

13. What is a counterproductive activity in the salon? _____

_____

14. Circle each correct answer. Successful stylists <u>do / *do not*</u> run themselves ragged; they <u>do / *do not*</u> eat, sleep, and drink beauty. They <u>do / do not</u> take care of their personal needs by spending time with family and friends, having hobbies, and enjoying recreational activities.

15. List three ways to show respect for others.

a) _____

b) _____

c) _____

16. Unscramble each term and then match it with its definition.

naotiostcrinpra   mfepnictsioer   eagm apln

_____   To put off until tomorrow what you can do today.

_____   The compulsion to do things perfectly.

_____   The conscious act of planning your life instead of just letting things happen.

17. When setting goals for yourself, how far ahead should you plan?

_____ Daily

_____ Weekly

_____ Yearly

_____ All of these answers are correct.

18. What must you first do to be successful? _____

19. It is ultimately your instructor's responsibility to make sure you learn what you need to in a course.

_____ True

_____ False

21. List the "rules" that will help take you down the road of success.

_____

_____

_____

_____

_____

_____

_____

_____

22. Discuss why it is important for you to continue to seek educational opportunities after you have completed school.

_____

_____

_____

23. What is the difference between motivation and self-management? _____

_____

_____

24. The best motivation for you to learn comes from an _____ to grow your skills as a professional.

25. What may happen to a person who is pursuing a career simply because others think it is the right career choice?

_____ a) The person will feel personally excited about her or his career choice.

_____ b) The person will never succeed in that career.

_____ c) The person may have trouble feeling motivated.

26. Define creativity. _____

_____

_____

27. Name four guidelines to follow to enhance your creativity.

a) _____

b) _____

c) _____

d) _____

28. What does "change your vocabulary" mean? _____

_____ What are some examples?

_____

29. Why is it important to avoid being self-critical? _____

_____

MANAGING YOUR CAREER

30. What is a mission statement? _____

_____

31. Write a personal mission statement that communicates who you are and what you want in life.

_____

_____

_____

_____

GOAL SETTING

32. What is the purpose of setting goals? _____

_____

33. Why is it important to map out your goals? _____

_____

34. Describe the difference between short-term goals and long-term goals.

_____

_____

35. List five short-term goals and five long-term goals and the actions required to achieve them.

SHORT-TERM GOALS	ACTION

LONG-TERM GOALS	ACTION

36. To stay on track, it is important to _____ your plan regularly.

37. Name two common goals a salon manager may set for a cosmetologist.

1) _____

2) _____

TIME MANAGEMENT

38. All people have a(n) _____, or natural rhythm, that helps them manage their time efficiently if they pay attention to it.

39. An average person spends _____ checking e-mail, surfing the Internet, or watching videos each day.

_____ a) one hour

_____ b) three hours

_____ c) four hours

_____ d) six hours

40. Read through the list of time-management techniques. Rate each as either a personal strength or an area you need to develop or improve.

_____

_____

_____

_____

Time-Management Techniques	Strength	Development Opportunity
Prioritizing tasks		
Designing my own time-management system		
Not taking on more than I can handle		
Learning problem-solving techniques		
Giving myself free time to regroup		
Taking notes of my thoughts and ideas		
Making schedules for my regular commitments		

Knowing personal energy levels throughout the day		
Rewarding myself for good work		
Using to-do lists to prioritize tasks and activities		
Including time for physical activity		
Scheduling a block of free time each day		
Making time management a habit		

41. What is the most important aspect of time management in the salon?

_____

_____

STUDY SKILLS

42. If you find studying overwhelming what can you do? _____

What can you do if you find your mind wanders in class? _____

_____

43. List the habits you can develop to improve your study skills.

_____

_____

_____

_____

_____

_____

_____

_____

_____

44. To achieve a goal, it is sometimes necessary to learn _____ skills.

45. Discuss why you think having a mentor might help you achieve your goals.

_____

_____

_____

_____

ETHICS

46. The moral principles by which we live and work are _____.

47. List the five professional behaviors that will show you are an ethical person.

a) _____

b) _____

c) _____

_____

d) _____

_____

e) _____

_____

48. Describe how to maintain your integrity. _____

_____

49. Nancy had a fight with her daughter before going to work at the salon; she relives the entire fight with her first client of the morning. What is Nancy demonstrating?

_____ a) Her honesty and directness with everyone because she speaks her mind

_____ b) Her ability to provide self-care by venting her feelings

_____ c) Her lack of discretion by sharing a personal issue with a client

PERSONALITY DEVELOPMENT AND ATTITUDE

50. What are the "ingredients" of a healthy, positive attitude? _____

_____

_____

51. What does it mean to be tactful? _____

_____

52. When is assertiveness no longer a positive quality? _____

_____

53. People are born with values and goals.

_____ True

_____ False

54. List five positive qualities of people who are effective communicators.

a) _____

b) _____

c) _____

d) _____

e) _____

55. Think about what having a "pleasing attitude" means to you personally and describe some ways you can work toward improving your attitude.

_____

_____

_____

_____

_____

_____

_____

CHAPTER 3 Your Professional Image

Date: _____

Rating: _____

Text Pages: 34–43

POINT TO PONDER:

"Every day you do one of two things: build health or produce disease in yourself." —**Adelle Davis**

WHY STUDY THE IMPORTANCE OF YOUR PROFESSIONAL IMAGE?

1. In your own words, explain why your professional image and the way you present yourself will affect your career in the beauty and wellness industry.

   _____

   _____

   _____

   _____

   _____

   _____

   _____

2. List the six components that help create a complete, professional image.

   _____

   _____

3. Explain in your own words why finding a salon that exhibits a professional image and working environment that suits your personal style is critical to your future career success.

   _____

   _____

   _____

_____

_____

_____

_____

_____

_____

_____

_____

4. A client is _____ likely to have confidence in a beauty professional who looks messy and wears outdated clothing.

_____ a) more

_____ b) less

BEAUTY AND WELLNESS

5. What does being well groomed begin with?_____

6. It is not necessary to do which of the following every day?

_____ a) Shower or bathe

_____ b) Be neat and clean

_____ c) Wear perfume

_____ d) Use deodorant

7. _____ is the daily maintenance of cleanliness by practicing good sanitary habits.

8. Working as a stylist behind the chair or doing makeup, nail care, or skin care means that you must be extremely meticulous about your hygiene.

_____ True

_____ False

9. One of the best ways to ensure that you always smell fresh and clean is to create a _____ to keep in your station or locker. List the items that should be included. _____

_____

10. While working in a salon, when is it necessary for you to wash your hands?

_____ a) Before you begin each service

_____ b) Whenever they are soiled

_____ c) After using the restroom

_____ d) All of these answers are correct.

11. What should you do if you smoke? _____

_____

_____

APPEARANCES COUNT

12. Which is an extremely important element of your professional image?

_____ a) Cell phone

_____ b) Expensive shears

_____ c) Well-groomed hair, skin, and nails

_____ d) Designer clothes

13. A cosmetologist who wears sunscreen regularly is demonstrating a commitment to professional beauty.

_____ True

_____ False

14. How often should you change your style? _____
_____ Why? _____

15. Why do many salons have a no-fragrance policy for staff members?

_____

_____

16. Salon owners and managers view _____, _____, and
_____ as being just as important as technical knowledge and skills.

17. What is one of the most vital aspects of good personal grooming?

_____

18. Explain why it is a good idea to invest in an apron or a smock. _____

_____

19. Noticing the ways in which other stylists are dressed will provide you with clues about a particular salon's _____ .

20. How can you make the best clothing choices that promote your career as a promising stylist? _____

21. Name three important considerations a professional stylist should remember when choosing clothing and accessories.

1) _____

2) _____

3) _____

22. What types of shoes are generally recommended? _____

_____

23. Makeup should be used to _____ your best features and _____ your less flattering ones.

24. It is safe to wear flip-flops when working around electricity and sharp implements as long as you are careful.

_____ True

_____ False

25. Which of the following examples demonstrates a positive attitude?

_____ a) Discussing salon policy with a coworker in front of a client

_____ b) Telling a client who drops in unexpectedly for a service that you will not see her without an appointment

_____ c) Finishing a service for a coworker who needs to leave work unexpectedly

_____ d) Calling in sick on the first warm day of spring

26. A professional is someone who remains _____ , even when under _____ .

YOUR PHYSICAL PRESENTATION

27. _____ is an important part of your physical presentation. Why? _____

_____

_____

28. List the guidelines for achieving and maintaining good work posture.

_____

_____

_____

_____

_____

29. Define ergonomics. _____

_____

_____

30. Give an example of fitting the job to the person in the salon. _____

_____

_____

31. The best way to avoid problems of the hands, wrists, shoulders, neck, back, feet, and legs is to _____ them from occurring in the first place.

32. The muscles and joints of the body can be injured by repetitive motions.

_____ True

_____ False

33. After your next practical service, analyze yourself to see if you do any of the following:

_____ Grip or squeeze implements too tightly.

_____ Bend the wrist up or down constantly when using your tools.

_____ Hold your arms away from your body as you work.

_____ Hold your elbows more than a 60-degree angle away from your body for extended periods of time.

_____ Bend forward and/or twist your body to get closer to your client.

34. What measures can you take to avoid these problems?

_____

_____

_____

_____

_____

_____

_____

_____

35. How can you counter the problem of working in an environment that has physical discomfort? _____

_____

36. You should always put your health first and the task at hand second.

_____ True

_____ False

4 Communicating for Success

Date: _____

Rating: _____

Text Pages: 44–64

POINT TO PONDER:

*"Wisdom is knowing when to speak your mind and when to mind your speech."—**Evangel***

WHY STUDY COMMUNICATING FOR SUCCESS?

1. List three things that effective communication skills will help.

1) _____

2) _____

3) _____

2. Give some examples of the ways in which trust, clarity, and loyalty will help cosmetologists build strong relationships with coworkers and clients.

_____

_____

_____

_____

_____

_____

_____

_____

_____

_____

_____

_____

_____

HUMAN RELATIONS

3. Once you get to know your clients really well, you will always be able to understand what they want.

_____ True

_____ False

4. The key to operating effectively in many professions is to _____.
Why is it especially true for cosmetologists? _____

_____

5. The best way to understand others is to begin with a firm understanding of

_____.

_____ a) the salon

_____ b) state law

_____ c) yourself

_____ d) your coworkers

6. What are good relationships built on? _____

7. List the emotions you feel when you feel secure. _____ List
the emotions you feel when you feel insecure. _____

8. How can you help people around you feel secure? _____

_____

9. List five ways to handle the ups and downs of human relations and explain what each one means to you.

Explanation

a) _____

_____

_____

_____

_____

b) _____

_____

_____

_____

c) _____

_____

_____

_____

_____

_____

_____

_____

d) _____

_____

_____

_____

e) _____

_____

_____

_____

_____

_____

10. What is one strategy for dealing with an aggressive client?

_____ a) Fight back

_____ b) Turn the other cheek

_____ c) Agree with him or her

_____ d) Refuse to continue the service

11. The deciding factor in whether a relationship is going to be rewarding or demoralizing is how much the other party is willing to give.

_____ True

_____ False

12. List the golden rules of effective human relations.

a) _____

b) _____

c) _____

d) _____

e) _____

_____

f) _____

g) _____

h) _____

i) _____

j) _____

k) _____

l) _____

COMMUNICATION BASICS

13. Define effective communication. _____

_____

14. Besides communicating with words, how else do people communicate? _____

_____

15. What is one of the most important communication encounters you will have with a client? _____

16. How should you act the first time you meet a client?

_____ a) Polite, friendly, aloof

_____ b) Polite, friendly, inviting

_____ c) Friendly, inviting, distant

_____ d) Casual, friendly, distant

17. Explain the steps you need to take to earn new clients' trust and loyalty.

a) _____

b) _____

c) _____

d) _____

e) _____

18. An intake form that is completed by every new client prior to service may also be called a _____ or a _____ .

19. In some cosmetology schools, the consultation card may be accompanied by a _____ . What is its purpose? _____

_____

_____

20. A new client should arrive approximately _____ ahead of her or his appointment to complete the consultation card.

THE CLIENT CONSULTATION (NEEDS ASSESSMENT)

21. What is the purpose of the client consultation? _____

_____

22. The client consultation is the single most important part of any service.

_____ True

_____ False

23. How often should a client consultation be performed?

_____ a) Never

_____ b) Every visit

_____ c) Every other visit

_____ d) Only for chemical services

24. A happy client means _____ for both you and the salon.

25. How can you ensure your time is well spent during the client consultation?

_____

26. What tools should you prepare for use in the client consultation?

a) _____

_____

b) _____

c) _____

27. An older client requests a hairstyle that is currently popular among teenagers, and you suspect it will not suit the client. What should you do?

_____

_____

_____

_____

_____

28. One key to a successful client consultation is making sure the client is _____ during the process.

29. Why is the intake form a valuable source of information about a client?

_____

_____

_____

_____

_____

_____

30. The following list is the 10-Step Consultation Method. In the space provided, list what you should do during each step.

10 Steps	**Action Taken**
1. Review	_____
	_____
2. Assess	_____
3. Preference	_____
	_____
	_____
	_____
	_____
	_____

4. Analyze _____

   _____

   _____

5. Lifestyle _____

   _____

   _____

   _____

6. Show and Tell _____

   _____

   _____

7. Suggest Options _____

   _____

   _____

   _____

   _____

   _____

8. Color Recom-
   mendations _____

   _____

   _____

9. Upkeep and
   Maintenance _____

   _____

   _____

   _____

10. Review the
    Consultation _____

   _____

   _____

   _____

31. Before making a recommendation to a client about a particular look or style, you must obtain the client's _____ to do so.

32. Which of the following is an example of a client's styling parameter?

_____ a) Hair type

_____ b) Ability

_____ c) Face shape

_____ d) All of these answers are correct.

33. Listening to a client and then repeating what you think a client is telling you, using your own words, is called _____.

34. Why do you think it is important to offer a client at least two additional services to complete or improve a style?

_____

_____

_____

_____

_____

35. Explain the three-step plan for making retailing recommendations to a client.

Step 1: _____

Step 2: _____

_____

Step 3: _____

36. At the end of a client needs assessment, you should not begin the service until the client _____ with your plan for proceeding.

37. At the conclusion of the service, what information should you record on the consultation card? _____

_____

SPECIAL ISSUES IN COMMUNICATION

38. Explain why tardy clients create a problem. _____

_____

_____

39. List ways in which tardy clients can be handled so that you do not lose their business or ruin your day's schedule.

a) _____

b) _____

_____

c) _____

_____

d) _____

_____

40. Decide which of the following is more likely to use the term client or guest when referring to its patrons. Write your answers on the lines that follow.

Day spa _____

Salon _____

Medical spa _____

41. What should you do when a scheduling mix-up occurs?

_____ Not admit that you or anyone in the salon made a mistake

_____ Argue with the client about who wrote the appointment down wrong

_____ Be polite and never argue the point of which one of you is correct

_____ Blame the salon receptionist and call the manager

42. A key to resolving a scheduling mix-up is to stay _____ and not make the situation personal.

43. Once you master all your hairstyling skills, you will never have an unhappy client.

_____ True

_____ False

44. Which of the following are appropriate ways of dealing with unhappy clients? (Check all that apply.)

_____ Find out why the client is unhappy.

_____ Do not change what the client dislikes until his or her next visit.

_____ Tactfully explain the reasons why you cannot make changes.

_____ Argue with the client or force your opinion.

_____ Allow the receptionist to handle the situation, so you can move on to your next client.

_____ Call on a more experienced stylist or salon manager for help.

45. To become a successful stylist, you should only work with clients who share your own age, style, and social background.

_____ True

_____ False

46. What is the best way to decide how to address new clients?

_____ a) Always use their first name.

_____ b) Use the honorific such as "Mrs. Brown" until clients tell you otherwise.

_____ c) Ask clients up front what they would like you to call them.

47. You do not need to follow the basic rules of professionalism when working with younger clients because most of them do not understand proper etiquette.

_____ True

_____ False

48. Why should you avoid using slang expressions when speaking with clients?

_____

_____

49. You are performing a consultation on a stylish, younger client when she uses a slang term to describe how she would like to look. You have no idea what the word means. What should you do next?

_____ a) Agree with whatever she said and hope it is not important.

_____ b) Explain that you are unfamiliar with that term, and ask her to explain what she means.

_____ c) Excuse yourself for a minute and try to find someone who knows what the term means.

50. It is unwise to become a client's counselor, career guide, parental sounding board, or motivational coach.

_____ True

_____ False

51. Which of the following conversation topics are considered neutral and appropriate for use with a client in the salon? (Check all that apply.)

_____ a) A new movie that was just released

_____ b) A scandal involving a local politician

_____ c) Your thoughts on teaching religion in school

_____ d) A new color line the salon is offering

_____ e) Your client's upcoming vacation

52. Think about interactions you have had in the past with other stylists when you have been the *client*. Name three examples of things you have liked about your relationship with a particular stylist. What made the interactions successful?

a) _____

_____

_____

_____

_____

_____

b) _____

_____

_____

c) _____

_____

_____

_____

IN-SALON COMMUNICATION

53. Behaving in a _____ is the first step in making meaningful, in-salon communication possible.

54. In the salon community, working closely for long hours with your coworkers, it is important to maintain _____ and remember that the salon is ultimately the place where you _____.

55. What guidelines should you keep in mind as you interact and communicate with fellow staffers?

a) _____

b) _____

c) _____

d) _____

e) _____

f) _____

g) _____

h) _____

56. Describe why you think participating in gossip can be as damaging to you as it is to the person about whom you are gossiping.

_____

_____

_____

_____

_____

_____

_____

57. Rewrite the following sentences to make them sound more professional.

a) Thanks for your help. _____

b) Sit in that chair by the window. _____

_____

c) Wow, your ends are really damaged! _____

_____

d) Yeah, so you are like saying you have no time for your hair. _____

_____

_____

58. It helps to remember that a manager is also a _____.

59. You disagree with a few of the rules in the salon where you work; it is OK for you to confide that to your clients.

_____ True

_____ False

60. What things should you strive for when dealing with your manager?

a) _____

b) _____

c) _____

d) _____

e) _____

f) _____

61. What kinds of salons conduct frequent and thorough employee evaluations?

_____

62. It is acceptable for you to ask to see the criteria on which you will be evaluated.

_____ True

_____ False

63. Should you rate yourself in the weeks and months ahead of your evaluation?
_____ Why? _____

64. Why do many professionals never see the evaluation meeting as a crucial communication opportunity to discuss future advancement with their managers?

_____

65. A self-evaluation demonstrates that you _____.

_____ do not trust your manager's assessment of your performance

_____ are planning to look for a new position elsewhere

_____ are serious about your growth and opportunities to improve

_____ do not think you are doing a good job

66. At the end of the meeting, you should _____

_____.

CHAPTER 5 Infection Control: Principles and Practices

Date: _____

Rating: _____

Text Pages: 65–107

POINT TO PONDER:

"One pound of learning requires ten pounds of common sense to apply it."—**Persian Proverb**

WHY STUDY INFECTION CONTROL?

1. Explain in your own words why it is important to study infection control.

   _____

   _____

   _____

   _____

   _____

2. Cosmetologists should understand the _____ of the cleaning and disinfecting products they use in the salon.

REGULATION

3. In regard to regulating the practice of cosmetology, what is the difference between federal agencies and state agencies? _____

   _____

   _____

   _____

   _____

4. What does OSHA stand for? _____

5. OSHA was created as part of the U.S. Department of Labor to _____

   _____

6. What is the purpose of the Hazard Communication Standard (HCS)?

_____

_____

7. Explain why you think OSHA's standards are important to you personally as a cosmetologist.

_____

_____

_____

_____

_____

8. Federal and state laws require manufacturers to supply a Material Safety Data Sheet (MSDS) only for those products that are potentially hazardous.

_____ True

_____ False

9. What does a Material Safety Data Sheet include? _____

_____

_____

_____

10. Federal and states laws require salons to obtain an MSDS for each product that is used in the salon.

_____ True

_____ False

11. It is the responsibility of each salon employee to _____ the information included on each MSDS and _____ they have done so by _____ a _____ sheet.

12. What does the Environmental Protection Agency (EPA) register?

_____

13. Define the term disinfectant. _____

_____

14. What two types of disinfectants are used in salons?

a) _____

b) _____

15. A(n) _____ may be harmful when used on certain tools in the salon.

16. As a rule of thumb, it is always better to use the most powerful disinfectant when cleaning up a spill in the salon.

_____ True

_____ False

17. By law, a disinfecting product must be:

_____ a) Used in the manner prescribed on its manufacturer's label.

_____ b) Approved for each specific use.

_____ c) Registered with the EPA.

_____ d) All of these answers are correct.

18. If you do not follow the instructions for mixing, contact time, and the type of surface the disinfecting product can be used on, you've broken federal law.

_____ True

_____ False

19. Why do state regulatory agencies exist? _____

_____

20. List four examples of state regulatory agencies.

a) _____

b) _____

c) _____

d) _____

21. State agencies, rules are enforced through _____ and investigations of consumer complaints.

22. Explain why it is important for a cosmetologist to understand and follow state laws and rules at all times.

_____

_____

_____

_____

_____

_____

23. A cosmetologist who is unsure about which disinfectant to use should:

_____ a) Choose the one that is most powerful.

_____ b) Use whatever is handy.

_____ c) Check state regulations.

_____ d) Scrub the instrument or surface with soap and water.

24. What is the difference between laws and rules?

_____

_____

_____

_____

_____

PRINCIPLES OF INFECTION

25. The invasion of body tissues by disease-causing pathogens is called

_____.

26. List the four types of potentially harmful organisms that are important in the practice of cosmetology.

a) _____

b) _____

c) _____

d) _____

27. Why are these organisms potentially harmful? _____

_____

28. It is appropriate for a cosmetologist to recommend a treatment to a client who has an abnormal condition, if the cosmetologist has personally had the same condition in the past and, therefore, understands how to treat it.

_____ True

_____ False

29. Use the following terms to complete the sentences below: fungicidal, clean, disinfection, virucidal, bactericidal.

a) _____ refers to something that is able to destroy viruses.

b) To _____ means to remove all visible debris, dirt, and many disease-causing germs by scrubbing using soap and water or detergent and water.

c) The process of _____ destroys many but not all microorganisms on nonporous surfaces.

d) To destroy a fungi, you would need to use something labeled as a

_____.

e) A product that is _____ is able to destroy bacteria.

30. Explain why a cosmetologist is obligated to provide safe services in the salon.

_____

_____

31. One-celled microorganisms with both plant and animal characteristics are known as _____. Where can they exist? _____

_____

32. The vast majority of bacteria which are completely harmless and do not produce disease are _____ organisms.

33. List some of the useful functions of nonpathogenic bacteria.

a) _____

b) _____

c) _____

d) _____

34. Pathogens are harmful because they may cause _____ or infection when they enter the body.

35. Match each term with its correct definition.

_____ 1. Germs

a) Poisonous substances produced by some microorganisms.

_____ 2. Microorganism

b) The transmission of infection from body fluids or blood through contact with a contaminated intermediate object (such as an implement or towel).

_____ 3. Parasite

c) One-celled microorganisms having both plant and animal characteristics. Some are harmful and some are harmless.

_____ 4. Bacteria

d) Organism of microscopic or submicroscopic size.

_____ 5. Virus

e) A medical condition that is spread from one person to another.

_____ 6. Infectious

f) Transmission of infection due to contact with blood or body fluids through touching, kissing, coughing, sneezing, and talking.

_____ 7. Toxin

g) An organism that lives on another organism.

_____ 8. Direct transmission

h) Synonyms for any disease-producing organism.

_____ 9. Indirect transmission

i) Microorganism capable of infecting almost all plants and animals that replicates only within cells of living hosts.

36. Match each of the following bacteria with its unique shape.

_____ 1. Cocci

a) Curved lines

_____ 2. Staphylococci

b) Spiral or corkscrew-shaped

_____ 3. Streptococci

c) Short, rod-shaped

_____ 4. Diplococci

d) Round-shaped

_____ 5. Bacilli

e) Grape-like clusters

_____ 6. Spirilla

f) Spherical

37. Pus-forming bacteria that cause abscesses, pustules, and boils are known as

_____.

38. Pus-forming bacteria that cause infections such as strep throat and blood poisoning are known as _____.

39. Diplococci are bacteria that cause diseases such as _____.

40. How do the following bacteria move about?

    a) Cocci   _____

    b) Bacilla   _____

    c) Spirilla   _____

41. A term that means "moving about" is _____ while the term _____ refers to movement under one's own power.

42. Unscramble these words and use them to complete the sentences below.

    briateac   sopotparlm   aticve   cniatvie

    _____ generally consist of an outer cell wall containing a liquid called _____. They manufacture their own food from the surrounding environment, give off waste products, and grow and reproduce. The life cycle of bacteria is made up of two distinct phases: the _____ stage, and the _____ or spore-forming stage.

43. During the active stage, bacteria:

    _____ a) Change color.

    _____ b) Die.

    _____ c) Grow.

    _____ d) Dry out.

44. The division of a bacteria cell is called _____. The cells that are formed are called _____.

45. What type of conditions do bacteria require to multiply?

    _____ a) Cool and dark

    _____ b) Warm and clean

    _____ c) Dark and dry

    _____ d) Warm and damp

46. What happens to bacteria in favorable conditions? _____
What happens in unfavorable conditions? _____

47. Why do certain bacteria, such as anthrax and tetanus bacilli, coat themselves with wax-like outer shells?

_____

48. What happens to bacteria when favorable conditions are restored?

_____

49. What occurs when body tissues are invaded by disease-causing or pathogenic bacteria? _____

50. _____ is the body's reaction to injury, irritation, or infection; it is characterized by _____, _____, _____, and _____.

51. What is pus?_____

_____

52. A local infection is one that is _____ to a particular part of the body.

53. Give an example of a local infection. _____

54. Staphylococci are among the most common human bacteria and are normally carried by what percentage of the population?

_____ a) 1/8

_____ b) 1/2

_____ c) 1/3

_____ d) 1/4

55. How is a staph infection most frequently transferred in the salon?

_____

_____

56. A MRSA infection can be _____ to cure.

_____ a) Easy

_____ b) Difficult

_____ c) Impossible

57. Staph infections occur most frequently in people who have _____ immune systems or who have had recent _____ procedures. The symptoms usually appear as skin infections such as:

_____.

58. It is possible for a client to have a staph infection without knowing it.

_____ True

_____ False

59. A disease that spreads from one person to another by contact is said to be contagious or _____.

60. List the more common contagious diseases that will prevent a cosmetologist from servicing a client. _____

_____

61. List twelve ways contagious diseases are commonly spread.

a) _____   g) _____

b) _____   h) _____

c) _____   i) _____

d) _____   j) _____

e) _____   k) _____

f) _____   l) _____

62. What are two differences between bacteria and viruses?

a) _____

_____

b) _____

_____

_____

63. Vaccinations prevent viruses from growing in the body, but are not available for all viruses.

_____ True

_____ False

64. Health authorities recommend that service providers in industries that have direct contact with the public, such as cosmetologists, receive a vaccination for _____.

65. The human papilloma virus (HPV) can infect the bottom of the _____.

66. A client who shows signs of an HPV infection should not receive a(n) _____ service.

67. Disease-causing microorganisms that are carried through the body in the blood or body fluids are called _____.

68. List nine ways disease-causing microorganisms can be spread inside the salon.

a) _____ f) _____

b) _____ g) _____

c) _____ h) _____

d) _____ i) _____

e) _____

69. It is against the law for a cosmetologist to _____ _____ _____, even if the client insists.

70. When is it appropriate for a cosmetologist to remove a callus on a client's foot?

_____ a) Upon the client's request

_____ b) As a routine part of a pedicure service

_____ c) Only if the callus causes the client discomfort

_____ d) None of these answers are correct.

71. List the three types of hepatitis that are of concern in the salon environment: _____.

72. Which of the three types of hepatitis is the most difficult to kill on a surface? _____

73. What does HIV stand for? _____

74. What does AIDS stand for? _____ What is AIDS? _____

75. Name some ways in which HIV is not transmitted. _____ _____

76. _____, which include molds, mildews, and yeasts, can produce _____ diseases such as ringworm.

77. Although it affects plants and inanimate objects, _____ does not cause human infections in the salon.

78. _____ is the most frequently encountered infection resulting from hair services. What does it affect? _____ _____ Whom does it mostly affect? _____

79. List the steps that should be followed to clean and disinfect clipper blades effectively.

1) _____

2) _____

80. Nail infections can be spread through _____ implements or when the natural nail is not properly _____ before applying an enhancement.

81. A(n) _____ nail infection is more common on the feet than on the hands.

82. _____ nail infections commonly occur on both the hands and the feet.

83. Nail services may cause which of the following infections if proper cleaning and disinfection procedures are not followed?

_____ a) Tinea barbae

_____ b) Tinea pedis

_____ c) Tinea capitis

84. _____ are organisms that grow, feed, and find shelter on or in another _____ and need that _____ to survive.

85. Name three external parasites that affect the human skin.

a) _____

b) _____

c) _____

86. Pathogenic bacteria or viruses or fungi can enter the body through:

a) _____

b) _____

c) _____

d) _____

e) _____

87. The body prevents and controls infections with:

a) _____

b) _____

c) _____

d) _____

88. Match each of the following terms with its definition.

_____ 1. Immunity

a) Both inherited and developed through healthy living.

_____ 2. Natural immunity

b) Ability to overcome disease through inoculation or exposure to allergens like pollen.

_____ 3. Acquired immunity

c) The body's ability to destroy and resist infection.

PRINCIPLES OF PREVENTION

89. Define the term decontamination. _____

_____

_____

90. Most salons use this method of decontamination: _____

_____ .

91. In some states, salons that also perform nail services must now use this method of decontamination: _____

92. The vast majority of pathogens and contaminants can be removed from the surfaces of tools and implements through proper cleaning.

_____ True

_____ False

93. If you are in a hurry to get to your next client, it is OK to use a disinfectant on an instrument and skip the step of cleaning it first.

_____ True

_____ False

94. List the three pathogens that disinfectants are able to destroy on nonporous surfaces: _____ .

95. Explain why disinfectants should not be used on human skin, hair, or nails.

_____

_____

_____

_____

96. Explain how sterilization is different from disinfection.

_____

_____

_____

_____

97. A high-pressure steam autoclave is the most effective method of

_____.

98. How often does the CDC require an autoclave to be tested to make sure it is functioning properly?

_____ Daily

_____ Weekly

_____ Twice a month

_____ Every two months

99. Currently, no states require salons to sterilize their tools and implements.

_____ True

_____ False

100. Disinfectants must be registered by the _____.

_____ CDC

_____ FDA

_____ EPA

101. What does it mean if a disinfectant has the word _concentrate_ on its label?

_____ It needs to be mixed with water before using.

_____ It is ready to use right out of the container.

_____ It is less potent than other types of disinfectants.

102. Define the term contact time. _____

_____

103. A disinfectant that is environmentally friendly can be _____ down the salon drain.

104. When compared to a hospital, a salon has a _____ infection risk.

_____ Higher

_____ Lower

105. Explain why you need to remove all dirt and other matter you can see on tools and implements before immersing them in disinfectant solution.

_____

_____

_____

_____

106. The label on a disinfectant product states "complete immersion." Explain what this means.

_____

_____

_____

107. _____, known as quats for short, are effective disinfectants for salon use, when used according to the product labeling instructions.

108. List six disadvantages of phenolic disinfectants.

a) _____

b) _____

c) _____

d) _____

e) _____

f) _____

109. Why should a cosmetologist know about accelerated hydrogen peroxide (AHP) ?

_____

_____

110. Any household bleach may be used as an effective disinfectant.

_____ True

_____ False

111. Name five disadvantages of using bleach as a disinfectant.

a) _____

b) _____

c) _____

d) _____

e) _____

112. Name two disinfectants that are unsafe for salon use.

a) _____

b) _____

113. Identify each of the following items used in a salon as either multiuse or single-use:

Nippers   _____

Cotton balls   _____

Permanent wave rods   _____

Combs   _____

Capes   _____

Pumice stones   _____

Wooden sticks   _____

114. According to state rules, how often should tools and equipment be cleaned and then disinfected? _____

115. In the salon, how should soiled linens and towels be stored until they can be properly laundered?

_____

116. Why is it good practice to clean doorknobs and handles daily?

_____

_____

117. Ultraviolet (UV) light units are effective for sterilizing implements.

_____ True

_____ False

118. A sanitizer is a cleaner and does not work as a disinfectant.

_____ True

_____ False

119. Why are liquid hand soaps preferred over bar soaps in the salon?

_____

UNIVERSAL PRECAUTIONS

120. What are Universal Precautions?

_____

_____

_____

121. Explain why strict infection control practices should be followed for every client.

_____

_____

_____

_____

122. A(n) _____ is contact with nonintact skin, blood, body fluid, and/or other potentially infectious materials during the performance of an employee's duties.

THE PROFESSIONAL SALON IMAGE

123. _____ is an important part of the salon routine and helps project a professional image to clients.

124. How often should you sweep hair off the floor of the salon?

_____ a) After every client

_____ b) Once a day

_____ c) As part of the closing routine

125. Explain why you think food should never be stored in the same refrigerator as salon products.

_____

_____

_____

_____

126. To maintain a professional image, try to avoid touching your _____, _____, or _____ during client services.

127. Name four important ways you can protect the health and safety of your salon clients.

a) _____

b) _____

c) _____

_____

d) _____

_____

6 General Anatomy and Physiology

CHAPTER

Date: _____

Rating: _____

Text Pages: 108–153

POINT TO PONDER:

"You will never change your life until you change something you do daily. The secret of your success is found in your daily routine."
—*John C. Maxwell*

WHY STUDY ANATOMY AND PHYSIOLOGY?

1. List the reasons a cosmetologist studies anatomy and physiology.

   a) _____

   b) _____

   c) _____

   _____

2. Before you begin this chapter, think about the areas of anatomy and physiology with which you are already familiar from past studies or experiences. Which body systems will it be most important for you to understand well?

   _____

   _____

   _____

   _____

   _____

ANATOMY, PHYSIOLOGY, AND YOU

3. As a cosmetologist, understanding the concept of human anatomy is primarily restricted to _____

   _____.

4. The study of human body structures you can see with the naked eye and how they are organized is called _____.

5. The study of structures that require a microscope to see is called _____.
_____ is the study of the functions and activities performed by the body's structures.

CELLS

6. The basic unit of all living things, from bacteria to plants and animals, including human beings is the _____.

7. The cells of all living things are composed of a substance called _____, a colorless, jelly-like substance.

8. Match each of the following terms with its definition.

_____ 1. binary fission

a) Chemical process through which cells are nourished and carry out their activities.

_____ 2. Metabolism

b) Dense active protoplasm, found at the center of the cell.

_____ 3. Histology

c) Protoplasm of the cell that surrounds the nucleus.

_____ 4. Nucleus

d) Cell division into two identical daughter cells.

_____ 5. Cytoplasm

e) Balloon that contains the protoplasm, allowing certain substances to pass through.

_____ 6. Cell membrane

f) Study of the many tiny structures found in living tissue; microscopic anatomy.

9. Cells have the ability to reproduce, providing new cells for the growth and replacement of worn or injured ones.

_____ True

_____ False

10. Most cells reproduce by dividing into two identical cells called _____. This process of cell reproduction is known as _____.

11. For cells to grow and reproduce, conditions must be _____, which include a(n):

a) _____

b) _____

c) _____

12. What occurs if conditions are unfavorable for cell growth and reproduction?

_____

13. What conditions are considered unfavorable for cell growth and reproduction?

_____

14. Identify the parts of the cell in the following illustration.

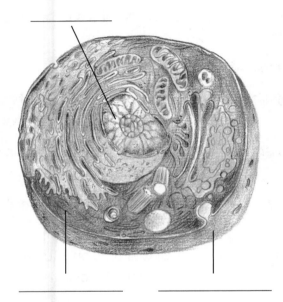

15. _____ is a chemical process that takes place in living organisms, whereby the cells are nourished and carry out their activities.

16. List and define the two phases of metabolism.

a) _____

_____

b) _____

_____

17. During which phase of metabolism is energy released that has been stored?

_____

18. During which phase of metabolism does the body store water, food, and oxygen? _____

19. Anabolism and catabolism are not carried out simultaneously.

_____ True

_____ False

TISSUES

20. A collection of similar cells that perform a particular function are _____.
Each collection has a specific function and can be recognized by its
_____ appearance.

21. How many types of tissue are there in the body? _____

22. _____ tissue is a protective covering on body surfaces.

_____ a) Connective

_____ b) Epithelial

_____ c) Muscular

_____ d) Nerve

23. _____ tissue contracts and moves the various parts of the body.

_____ a) Connective

_____ b) Epithelial

_____ c) Muscular

_____ d) Nerve

_____ e) Liquid

24. _____ tissue serves to support, protect, and bind together other tissues
of the body.

_____ a) Connective

_____ b) Epithelial

_____ c) Muscular

_____ d) Nerve

_____ e) Liquid

25. Tissues such as blood and lymph that carry food, waste products, and
hormones through the body are _____.

_____ a) connective

_____ b) epithelial

_____ c) muscular

_____ d) nerve

_____ e) liquid

26. _____ tissues carry messages to and from the brain and control and coordinate all bodily functions.

_____ a) Connective

_____ b) Epithelial

_____ c) Muscular

_____ d) Nerve

_____ e) Liquid

27. List examples of connective tissue: _____

_____

28. List examples of epithelial tissue: _____

_____

ORGANS AND BODY SYSTEMS

29. Groups of tissues designed to perform a specific function are _____.

30. _____ are groups of bodily organs acting together to perform one or more functions. There are _____ major systems.

31. Give the functions of the following systems.

a) Circulatory: _____

b) Digestive: _____

c) Endocrine: _____

_____

d) Excretory: _____

e) Integumentary: _____

_____

f) Lymphatic _____

_____

g) Muscular: _____

h) Nervous: _____

i) Reproductive: _____

_____

j) Respiratory: _____

k) Skeletal: _____

THE SKELETAL SYSTEM

32. _____ is the study of anatomy, structure, and functions of the bones. What prefix used in many medical terms means "bone"? _____

33. The skeletal system is composed of _____ bones that vary in size and shape and are connected by _____ and _____ joints.

34. How many bones does a newborn have? _____ Why does this number decrease as we grow older? _____

_____

35. Other than bone, what is the hardest tissue in the body? _____

_____

36. List the five primary functions of the skeletal system.

   a) _____

   b) _____

   c) _____

   _____

   d) _____

   e) _____

   _____

37. A _____ is the connection between two or more bones of the skeleton.

38. The two types of joints are _____.

39. Provide examples of movable joints: _____

40. Provide examples of immovable joints: _____

41. How many moveable and semi-moveable joints does the human body have?

_____

42. The skull is divided into two parts: the _____ and the _____, which is made up of _____ bones.

43. The cranium is made up of:

_____ a) 8 bones

_____ b) 10 bones

_____ c) 2 bones

_____ d) 14 bones

44. Match each of the following bones of the cranium with its description.

_____ 1. Parietal   a) Forms the forehead

_____ 2. Occipital   b) Hindmost bone of the skull

_____ 3. Frontal   c) Form the sides of the head in the ear region

_____ 4. Temporal   d) Form the sides and crown of the cranium

45. Match each of the following bones of the face with its description.

_____ 1. Nasal   a) Small, thin bones located at the front
             inner wall

_____ 2. Lacrimal   b) Lower jawbone, largest and strongest
             of the face

_____ 3. Zygomatic   c) Form the bridge of the nose

_____ 4. Maxillae   d) Bones of the upper jaw

_____ 5. Mandible   e) Form the prominence of the cheeks

46. Match each of the following bones of the neck, chest, shoulder, and back with its description.

_____ 1. Hyoid   a) U-shaped bone at the base of the tongue

_____ 2. Cervical vertebrae b) The chest; elastic, bony cage

_____ 3. Thorax   c) Shoulder blades

_____ 4. Ribs   d) Collarbone

_____ 5. Scapula   e) Breastbone

_____ 6. Sternum   f) Twelve pairs of bones forming the wall of
             the thorax

_____ 7. Clavicle   g) Seven bones that form the top part of the
             vertebral column

47. The smaller bone in the forearm on the same side as the thumb is the:

_____ a) Humerus

_____ b) Radius

_____ c) Carpus

_____ d) Ulna

48. The uppermost and largest bone of the arm is the:

_____ a) Humerus

_____ b) Radius

_____ c) Carpus

_____ d) Ulna

49. Another name for the wrist, a flexible joint composed of a group of eight small, irregular bones, is the _____.

50. The inner, large bone of the forearm, which is attached to the wrist and located on the side of the little finger, is the _____.

51. The _____ are the bones of the palm of the hand, and the phalanges are the bones in the fingers, also called _____.

52. Match each of the following terms with its description.

_____ 1. Femur   a) Accessory bone; forms the kneecap joint

_____ 2. Tibia   b) Heavy, long bone; forms the leg above the knee

_____ 3. Fibula   c) Smaller of two bones, forms the leg below the knee

_____ 4. Patella   d) Ankle bone of the foot

_____ 5. Talus   e) Larger of two bones that form the leg below the knee

53. The foot is made up of _____ bones, subdivided into three categories:

a) _____

b) _____

c) _____

THE MUSCULAR SYSTEM

54. Define the muscular system. _____

_____

55. The study of the structure, function, and diseases of the muscles is
_____ . The human body has over _____ muscles, which are
responsible for approximately _____ of the body's weight.

56. List the three types of muscular tissue.

a) _____

b) _____

c) _____

57. _____ muscles, also called _____ muscles, are attached to the bones
and are voluntary, or controlled by the will.

58. _____ muscles, or _____ muscles, are involuntary and function
automatically, without conscious will.

59. _____ muscle is the involuntary muscle that is the heart.

60. List the two functions of the striated muscles. _____

_____

61. Where are nonstriated muscles found? _____

_____

62. Cardiac muscle is found in several parts of the body besides the heart?

_____ True

_____ False

63. Name the three parts of the muscle and define each part.

a) _____

b) _____

_____

c) _____

64. In which directions is pressure applied to the muscle during massage?

_____

65. List seven ways in which muscular tissue can be stimulated.

a) _____

b) _____

c) _____

d) _____

e) _____

f) _____

g) _____

66. The broad muscle that covers the top of the skull is the _____.
It consists of two parts: the _____ and the _____.

67. The muscle that draws the scalp backward is the _____ .

68. The _____ muscle of the scalp raises the eyebrows, draws the scalp forward, and causes wrinkles across the forehead.

69. What tendon connects the occipitalis and the frontalis? _____

70. Match each of the muscles of the ear to its description.

_____ 1. Auricularis superior   a) Muscle behind the ear that draws the ear backward

_____ 2. Auricularis anterior   b) Muscle above the ear that draws the ear upward

_____ 3. Auricularis posterior   c) Muscle in front of the ear that draws the ear forward

71. The three muscles of the ear have no function.

_____ True

_____ False

72. The masseter and the temporalis muscles coordinate the opening and closing of the mouth and are sometimes referred to as the _____.

73. In addition to the masseter and the temporalis muscles, what other muscles aid with mastication?

a) _____

b) _____

74. The broad muscle extending from the chest and shoulder muscles to the side of the chin is the _____.
What does this muscle do? _____

75. Which muscle of the neck lowers and rotates the head?

_____

76. The muscle located beneath the frontalis that draws the eyebrow down is the:

_____ a) Corrugator

_____ b) Orbicularis oculi

_____ c) Orbicularis oris

_____ d) Procerus

77. The muscle that covers the bridge of the nose, lowers the eyebrows, and causes wrinkles across the bridge of the nose is the:

_____ a) Corrugator

_____ b) Orbicularis oculi

_____ c) Orbicularis oris

_____ d) Procerus

78. The muscle that forms the ring of the eye socket, closing the eye is the.

_____ a) Corrugator

_____ b) Orbicularis oculi

_____ c) Orbicularis oris

_____ d) Procerus

79. Match each of the following muscles of the mouth with its description.

_____ 1. Buccinator

_____ 2. Depressor labii inferioris

_____ 3. Levator anguli oris

_____ 4. Levator labii superioris

_____ 5. Mentalis

_____ 6. Orbicularis oris

_____ 7. Risorius

a) Muscle that elevates the lower lip and raises and wrinkles the skin of the chin

b) Muscles extending from the zygomatic bone to the angle of the mouth that elevate the lip

c) Flat muscle of the cheek between the upper and lower jaw that compresses the cheeks and expels air between the lips

d) Muscle that raises the angle of the mouth and draws it inward

e) Muscle of the mouth that draws the corner of the mouth out and back

f) Muscle extending alongside the chin that pulls down the corner of the mouth

g) A muscle surrounding the lower lip; lowers the lower lip and draws it to one side

_____ 8. Triangularis

h) Flat band around the upper and lower lips that compresses, contracts, puckers, and wrinkles the lips

_____ 9. Zygomaticus

i) Muscle surrounding the upper lip; elevates the upper lip and dilates the nostrils

80. A person uses how many muscles to control his or her expressions?_____

81. The broad, flat superficial muscle covering the back of the neck and upper and middle region of the back is the:

_____ a) Pectoralis major

_____ b) Serratus anterior

_____ c) Latissimus dorsi

_____ d) Trapezius

82. The muscle that covers the back of the neck and upper middle region of the back and rotates and controls the swinging movements of the arm is the:

_____ a) Pectoralis major

_____ b) Serratus anterior

_____ c) Latissimus dorsi

_____ d) Trapezius

83. The muscles of the chest that assist the swinging movements of the arm are the:

_____ a) Pectoralis major

_____ b) Serratus anterior

_____ c) Latissimus dorsi

_____ d) Trapezius

84. The muscle of the chest that assists in breathing and in raising the arm is the:

_____ a) Pectoralis major

_____ b) Serratus anterior

_____ c) Latissimus dorsi

_____ d) Trapezius

85. What are the three principal muscles of the shoulders and upper arms?

_____

86. Match each of the following muscles with its description.

_____ 1. Biceps   a) Muscles that straighten the wrist, hand, and fingers to form a straight line

_____ 2. Deltoids   b) Muscle producing the contour of the front and inner side of the upper arm

_____ 3. Triceps   c) Muscles that turn the hand inward so that the palm faces downward

_____ 4. Extensors   d) Muscle of the forearm that rotates the radius outward and the palm upward

_____ 5. Flexors   e) Large triangular muscle covering the shoulder joints

_____ 6. Pronators   f) Extensor muscles of the wrist; involved in bending the wrist

_____ 7. Supinator   g) Large muscle that covers the entire back of the upper arm and extends the forearm

87. What is the difference between the abductor and adductor muscles?

_____

_____

_____

_____

88. The muscle that bends the foot up and extends the toes is the:

_____ a) Peroneus brevis

_____ b) Tibialis anterior

_____ c) Peroneus longus

_____ d) Extensor digitorum longus

89. The muscle that covers the front of the shin and bends the foot upward and inward is the:

_____ a) Peroneus brevis

_____ b) Tibialis anterior

_____ c) Peroneus longus

_____ d) Extensor digitorum longus

90. The muscle that covers the outside of the calf and inverts the foot, turns it outward is the:

_____ a) Peroneus brevis

_____ b) Tibialis anterior

_____ c) Peroneus longus

_____ d) Extensor digitorum longus

91. The muscle that originates at the upper portion of the fibula and bends the foot down is the:

_____ a) Gastrocnemius

_____ b) Soleus

_____ c) Peroneus brevis

_____ d) Peroneus longus

92. The muscle attached to the lower rear surface of the heel that pulls the foot down is the:

_____ a) Gastrocnemius

_____ b) Soleus

_____ c) Peroneus brevis

_____ d) Peroneus logus

93. Name the muscles of the feet.

a) _____

b) _____

c) _____

d) _____

THE NERVOUS SYSTEM

94. The system that is exceptionally well-organized and is responsible for coordinating all of the many activities that are performed inside and outside the body is the _____.

95. _____ is the scientific study of the structure, function, and pathology of the nervous system.

96. Every square inch (2.5 cm) of human body is supplied with fine fibers know as _____.

97. Why is it important for a cosmetologist to understand how the nervous system works? _____

_____

_____

98. What are the principal components of the nervous system?

_____

99. List the three main subdivisions of the nervous system.

a) _____

b) _____

c) _____

100. Name the subdivision of the nervous system identified by each of the following descriptions.

_____ System of nerves that connect the outer parts of the body to the central nervous system

_____ Consists of the brain, spinal cord, spinal nerves, and cranial nerves

_____ Controls the involuntary muscles

_____ Regulates the action of the smooth muscles, glands, blood vessels, and heart

_____ Controls consciousness and many mental activities, voluntary functions of the five senses, and voluntary muscle

_____ Carries impulses, or messages, to and from the central nervous system

101. The _____ is the largest and most complex nerve tissue in the body, is contained in the _____ , and weighs a little less than _____ pounds on average.

102. The portion of the central nervous system that originates in the brain, extends down to the lower extremity of the trunk, and is protected by the spinal column is the _____ . How many pairs of spinal nerves extend from it? _____

103. A _____ , also called a nerve cell, is the primary structural unit of the nervous system and is composed of a _____ and _____ .

104. Tree-like branchings of nerve fibers extending from the nerve cell that receive impulses from other neurons are _____ ; the _____ sends impulses away from the cell body to the other neurons, glands, or muscles.

105. The whitish cords made up of bundles of nerve fibers held together by connective tissue through which impulses are transmitted are _____. Where do they have their origin? _____

106. There are _____ types of nerves: _____, which carry impulses or messages from the sense organs to the brain, and _____, which carry impulses from the brain to the muscles.

107. The two types of nerves are also known as _____ nerves and _____ nerves.

108. The sensations of touch, cold, heat, sight, hearing, taste, smell, pain, and pressure are experienced by the _____ nerves.

109. How does information about different sensations reach the brain?

_____

_____

110. The impulses that produce movement are transmitted by the _____ nerves.

111. What is a reflex and how does it work?

_____

_____

_____

_____

_____

112. Which of the cranial nerves is the largest? _____ List the two additional names for this nerve: _____. What is the purpose of this nerve: _____

_____.

113. List the three branches of the fifth cranial nerve and their function.

a) _____   _____

_____

_____

b) _____   _____

_____

c) _____   _____

114. The fifth cranial nerve branches into many different nerves. Explain which part of the face each of the following nerves affect.

a) Auriculotemporal nerve: _____

_____

b) Infraorbital nerve: _____

_____

c) Infratrochlear nerve: _____

d) Mental nerve: _____

e) Nasal nerve: _____

f) Supraorbital nerve: _____

g) Supratrochlear nerve: _____

h) Zygomatic nerve: _____

115. The motor nerve of the face is the _____ cranial nerve.

116. List the most important branches of the facial nerve.

a) _____

b) _____

c) _____

d) _____

e) _____

f) _____

117. What does the greater occipital nerve affect?

_____ a) Muscles behind the ear

_____ b) Scalp and top of the head

_____ c) Parotid gland

_____ d) Breastbone

118. Which nerve controls the movement of the neck and shoulder muscles and is affected during a massage given as part of a facial? _____

_____

119. The principal nerves supplying the superficial parts of the arm and hand are the _____, _____, _____, and the _____.

120. Identify the nerves of the arm and hand in the illustration.

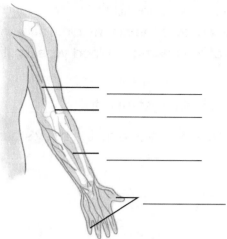

121. The nerve that supplies impulses to the knee, the muscles of the calf, the skin of the leg, and the sole, heel, and underside of the toes is the _____.

122. Match each of the following terms with its definition.

_____ 1. Common peroneal nerve

a) Extends down the leg; supplies impulses to the muscles and skin of the leg.

_____ 2. Deep peroneal nerve

b) Extends from behind the knee to wind around the head of the fibula to the front of the leg.

_____ 3. Superficial peroneal nerve

c) Extends down to the front of the leg; supplies to the muscles and skin on top of the foot and adjacent sides of the first and second toe.

123. Which nerve supplies impulses to the skin on the outer side and back of the foot and leg?

_____ a) Saphenous

_____ b) Sural

_____ c) Dorsal

_____ d) Tibial

124. Which nerve supplies impulses to the toes, foot, and muscles of the skin and the leg?

_____ a) Saphenous

_____ b) Sural

_____ c) Dorsal

_____ d) Tibial

THE CIRCULATORY SYSTEM

125. The circulatory system, also referred to as the _____ or _____ system, controls the steady circulation of the blood through the body by means of the heart and blood vessels. It consists of the _____.

126. The purpose of the vascular system is to _____.

127. Which of the following is referred to as the body's pump?

_____ a) Cells

_____ b) Lungs

_____ c) Heart

_____ d) Veins

128. Match each of the parts of the heart with its description.

_____ 1. Atrium   (a) Structures between the chambers that allow the blood to flow in only one direction

_____ Ventricle   (b) Upper, thin-walled chambers on the right and left

_____ Valves   (c) Lower, thick-walled chambers on the right and left

129. Two systems circulate the blood constantly from the time it leaves the heart until it returns. _____ sends the blood from the heart to the lungs to be purified, while _____ carries the blood from the heart throughout the body and back to the heart.

130. Explain how pulmonary and systemic circulation work.

a) _____

b) _____

_____

c) _____

_____

d) _____

e) _____

_____

f) _____

131. The three categories of blood vessels are _____, _____, and _____.

132. Match each of the following terms with its description.

_____ 1. Arteries   a) Tiny, thin walled blood vessels that connect the smaller arteries to the veins

_____ 2. Capillaries   b) Thin-walled blood vessels that are less elastic

_____ 3. Veins   c) Thick-walled, muscular, flexible tubes

_____ 4. Venules   d) Small arteries that deliver blood to capillaries

_____ 5. Arterioles   e) Small vessels that connect the capillaries to the veins

133. Identify the main parts of the heart shown in the following illustration.

To upper part of body

134. What is blood? _____

135. There are approximately _____ pints of blood in the human body, contributing to about _____ of the body's weight. Blood is approximately _____ water with a normal temperature of _____ °F.

136. Match each of the following terms with its description.

_____ 1. Red blood cells   a) Contribute to the blood-clotting process

_____ 2. Hemoglobin   b) Fluid part of the blood

_____ 3. White blood cells   c) Produced in the red bone marrow

_____ 4. Platelets   d) Perform the function of destroying disease-causing microorganisms

_____ 5. Plasma   e) Complex iron protein that binds to oxygen

137. What five critical functions does blood perform?

a) _____

b) _____

_____

c) _____

_____

d) _____

_____

e) _____

_____

138. The arteries located on either side of the neck that are the main sources of blood supply to the head, face, and neck are the _____ arteries.

139. The internal carotid artery supplies blood to the _____

_____.

140. The external carotid artery supplies blood to the _____

_____.

141. The artery that supplies blood to the lower region of the face, mouth, and nose is the:

_____ a) Facial artery

_____ b) Angular artery

_____ c) Superficial temporal artery

_____ d) Superior labial artery

142. The artery that supplies blood to the upper lip and region of the nose is the:

_____ a) Facial artery

_____ b) Angular artery

_____ c) Superficial temporal artery

_____ d) Superior labial artery

143. The artery that supplies blood to the skin and masseter is the:

_____ a) Parietal artery

_____ b) Transverse facial artery

_____ c) Middle temporal artery

_____ d) Anterior auricular artery

144. The popliteal artery divides into two separate arteries; one of these is called the:

_____ a) Parietal artery

_____ b) Transverse facial artery

_____ c) Anterior tibial artery

_____ d) Anterior auricular artery

145. The _____ and _____ arteries are the main blood supply for the arms and hands.

146. Identify the arteries of the arm and hand in the following illustration:

THE LYMPHATIC/IMMUNE SYSTEM

147. The lymphatic/immune system is closely related to the _____ system and consists of the _____ and other structures.

148. The purpose of lymph is to _____ .

149. List the primary functions of the lymphatic/immune system.

a) _____

b) _____

c) _____

d) _____

THE ENDOCRINE SYSTEM

150. The endocrine system is made up of a group of specialized glands that affect:

a) _____

b) _____

c) _____

d) _____

151. What are glands? _____

_____

152. Name the two main types of glands and their functions.

a) _____

_____

b) _____

_____

153. What are hormones? _____

_____

154. Give three examples of hormones.

a) _____

b) _____

c) _____

155. The thyroid gland plays a role in which of the following?

_____ a) Sexual development

_____ b) Blood pressure

_____ c) Metabolism

_____ d) Digesting carbohydrates

156. The pancreas plays a role in which of the following?

_____ a) Sexual development

_____ b) Blood pressure

_____ c) Metabolism

_____ d) Digesting carbohydrates

157. The pineal gland plays a role in which of the following?

_____ a) Sexual development

_____ b) Blood pressure

_____ c) Metabolism

_____ d) Digesting carbohydrates

THE DIGESTIVE SYSTEM

158. The digestive system is responsible for _____

_____ .

159. How long does the entire food digestion process take? _____

160. What do digestive enzymes do?_____

_____

THE EXCRETORY SYSTEM

161. The _____ is responsible for purifying the body by eliminating waste.

162. Match each organ of the excretory system with its function.

_____ 1. Kidneys | a) Eliminates decomposed and undigested food

_____ 2. Liver | b) Eliminates waste containing perspiration

_____ 3. Skin | c) Excrete waste containing urine

_____ 4. Large intestine | d) Discharges waste containing bile

_____ 5. Lungs | e) Exhale carbon dioxide

THE RESPIRATORY SYSTEM

163. The respiratory system enables breathing or _____ and consists of the lungs and air passages.

164. The spongy tissues composed of microscopic cells in which inhaled air is exchanged for carbon dioxide during one breathing cycle are the _____ .

165. The _____ is a muscular wall that separates the thorax from the abdominal region and helps control breathing.

166. During _____ or breathing in, oxygen is passed into the blood; during _____ or breathing outward, carbon dioxide is expelled from the lungs.

167. How long can a person survive without oxygen? _____

THE INTEGUMENTARY SYSTEM

168. The _____ is made up of the skin and its various accessory organs such as the _____, _____, _____,

and _____.

169. How many dead skin cells does a person's body shed every minute?

_____ a) 500 to 1,000

_____ b) 5, 000 to 15,000

_____ c) 30,000 to 40,000

_____ d) 50,000 to 75,000

THE REPRODUCTIVE SYSTEM

170. The organs on the female reproductive system include the _____

_____.

171. The organs on the male reproductive system include the _____

_____.

172. What are some unwanted results that may be caused by fluctuating female or male hormones? _____

_____

CHAPTER 7 Skin Structure, Growth, and Nutrition

Date: _____

Rating: _____

Text Pages: 154–173

POINT TO PONDER

"To do a common thing uncommonly well brings success."
—Henry John Heinz

WHY STUDY SKIN STRUCTURE, GROWTH, AND NUTRITION?

1. Clients with certain skin conditions should be referred to a medical professional for treatment.

   _____ True

   _____ False

2. Describe in your own words why you think it is necessary for a cosmetologist to stay on top of changes in skin care.

   _____

   _____

   _____

   _____

   _____

ANATOMY OF THE SKIN

3. The medical branch of science that deals with the study of skin and its nature, structure, functions, diseases, and treatment is called _____.

4. A _____ is a physician engaged in the science of treating the skin, its structures, functions, and diseases.

5. Some skin symptoms may be a sign of internal _____.

6. By law, in all states cosmetologists may clean skin, preserve the health of skin, and beautify skin.

_____ True

_____ False

7. An _____ is a cosmetologist who specializes in the cleansing, preservation of health, and beautification of the skin and body.

8. This professional may diagnose an abnormal skin condition:

_____ Esthetician

_____ Cosmetologist

_____ Nutritionist

_____ Dermatologist

9. The skin is the largest organ of the body.

_____ True

_____ False

10. The skin is our only barrier against the environment and protects

a) _____

b) _____

c) _____

d) _____

11. Healthy skin is _____

_____.

12. List the appendages of the skin.

a) _____

b) _____

c) _____

d) _____

13. The thinnest skin is found on the _____, and the thickest skin is found on the _____.

14. Explain how a callus forms and give an example of how one may occur.

_____

_____

_____

15. When is it appropriate to remove a callus in the salon? _____

_____

16. Explain the difference between the skin of the scalp and the skin elsewhere on the human body. _____

_____

_____

17. The skin is composed of two main divisions, the _____ and the

_____.

18. The _____ is the outermost layer of the skin and is also called the

_____. It is the thinnest layer of skin and forms a _____ for the body.

19. Name the five layers that make up the epidermis.

a) _____

b) _____

c) _____

d) _____

e) _____

20. The basal cell layer is also referred to as the _____ and is the deepest layer of the epidermis. It is the _____ of the epidermis and is responsible for the growth of the _____.

21. The basal cell layer also contains special cells called _____, which produce a dark skin pigment called _____.

22. The _____, also referred to as the stratum spinosum, is the layer where the process of skin cell shedding begins.

23. The stratum granulosum, or _____, consists of cells that are almost dead and are pushed to the surface to replace cells that are shed from the skin surface layer.

24. The _____ is the clear, transparent layer just under the skin surface, and the _____ is the outer layer of the epidermis.

25. Identify the layers of the skin illustrated below:

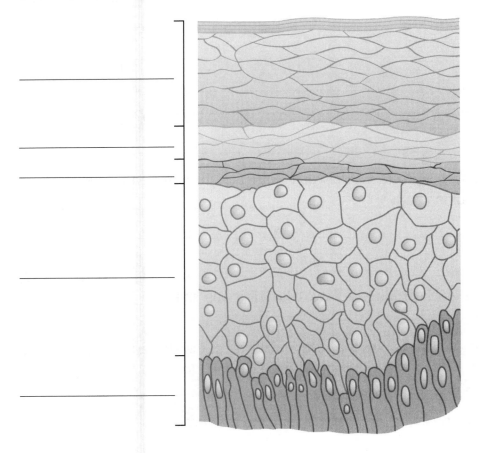

26. How thick is the skin? _____

27. The _____ is the underlying or inner layer of the skin and is made up of two layers: the _____ and the _____.

28. Describe what causes goose bumps or goose flesh.

_____

_____

_____

29. Which layer is the outer layer of the dermis, located directly beneath the epidermis? _____

30. Which layer is the deeper layer of the dermis that supplies the skin with oxygen and nutrients? _____

31. The reticular layer contains the following structures within its network:

a) _____

b) _____

c) _____

d) _____

e) _____

f) _____

g) _____

32. Where is the subcutaneous or fatty layer found? _____

33. This fatty tissue is also called _____ or _____ tissue and varies in thickness according to _____, _____, and _____

_____.

34. What are the functions of fat? _____

_____

35. _____ supplies nutrients and oxygen to the skin. _____, the clear fluids of the body that resemble blood plasma, bathe the skin cells, _____ and _____, and have immune functions that help protect the skin and body against diseases.

36. Which part of the skin does a cosmetologist or esthetician work on in the salon?

_____ Stratum corneum

_____ Stratum lucidum

_____ Stratum spinosum

_____ Stratum germinativum

37. The skin contains the surface endings of the following nerve fibers:

a) _____

b) _____

c) _____

38. _____ nerve fibers react to heat, cold, touch, pressure, and pain.

39. _____ nerve fibers are distributed to the arrector pili muscles.

40. Which nerve fibers are part of the autonomic nervous system, regulate the excretion of perspiration from the sweat glands, and control the flow of sebum?

_____

41. The nerve endings that provide the body with the sense of touch are housed in the _____ layer of the dermis.

42. The color of the skin depends primarily on _____, which are tiny grains of pigment deposited into cells in the _____ of the epidermis and papillary layers of the dermis.

43. Name and describe the two types of melanin.

a) _____

b) _____

44. Skin color is a _____ trait, and your _____ determine the amount and type of pigment your body produces.

45. Why do you need to use sunscreen if melanin helps protect your body from the sun? _____

_____

_____

46. What are the two structures that skin gets its strength, form, and flexibility from?

a) _____

b) _____

47. What are some causes of wrinkles and sagging skin?

_____

_____

_____

48. According to scientists, most signs of aging are caused by _____

_____.

49. When does the skin first begin to age? _____ Why?

_____

50. The skin contains two types of duct glands, _____ _____ and _____, that extract materials from the blood to form new substances.

51. The sudoriferous glands excrete

_____ a) Fragrance

_____ b) Water

_____ c) Oil

_____ d) Sweat

52. The sweat glands regulate _____ and help to eliminate _____ from the body. They are found on all parts of the body, but are more numerous on the _____.

53. The excretion of sweat is controlled by the _____, and normally, _____ of liquids containing salts are eliminated daily through sweat pores.

54. The sebaceous or oil glands of the skin are connected to the _____. _____ is a fatty or oil secretion that lubricates the skin and preserves the softness of the hair.

55. Sebaceous glands are not found on the

_____ a) Scalp

_____ b) Palms

_____ c) Face

_____ d) Knees

56. When the sebum hardens and the duct becomes clogged, a pore impaction or _____ is formed.

57. Name two functions of sebum.

a) _____

b) _____

58. List the principle functions of the skin.

a) _____   d) _____

b) _____   e) _____

c) _____   f) _____

59. Why do you think touch is one of the first senses to develop in the human body?

_____

_____

_____

_____

_____

60. Cosmetic products are designed to penetrate the epidermis.

_____ True

_____ False

NUTRITION AND MAINTAINING SKIN HEALTH

61. Name the six classes of nutrients necessary for the health of the body.

a) _____ d) _____

b) _____ e) _____

c) _____ f) _____

62. The body makes all of the nutrients it needs.

_____ True

_____ False

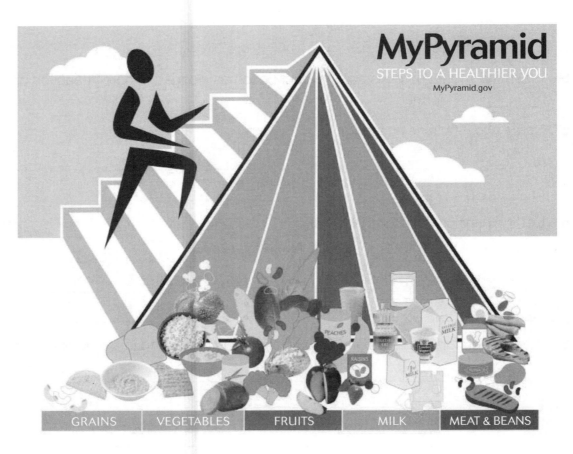

63. Based on the USDA food pyramid, what are the best types of vegetables for a person to eat each day? _____

_____

64. List some ways meat should be prepared according to the USDA food pyramid.

_____

65. Fruit juices are as beneficial as eating fresh, frozen, canned, or dried fruits according to the USDA food pyramid.

_____ True

_____ False

66. Seeds and nuts provide another source of protein in your diet according to the USDA food pyramid.

_____ True

_____ False

67. To maintain a balanced diet, a person should eat a(n) _____ of foods.

68. A healthy diet includes more _____, _____, and _____ products.

69. A healthy diet includes less _____, _____, and _____.

70. Prepared or processed foods contain _____ and modified _____.

71. A healthy diet should be balanced by the right amount of _____.

72. Explain what information is found on a food label.

_____

_____

73. What does RDA stand for? _____

74. Vitamins are nutritional supplements, not cosmetic ingredients.

_____ True

_____ False

75. Some vitamins have a positive effect on the skin when taken by mouth.

_____ True

_____ False

76. Match the following vitamin with its effect on healthy skin:

_____ Vitamin A   a) Promotes the healthy and rapid healing of skin

_____ Vitamin C   b) Aids in the health, function, and repair of skin cells

_____ Vitamin D   c) Helps protect the skin from harmful effects of UV light

_____ Vitamin E   d) Aids in and speeds up the healing process of the body

77. The best way of making sure your body gets the nutrients it needs each day is to:

_____ a) Take a nutritional supplement

_____ b) Improve your diet

_____ c) Avoid all fats

_____ d) Drink more water

78. Water comprises _____ of the body's weight.

79. The amount of water each person needs depends on:

a) _____

b) _____

80. Drinking pure water is essential to the health of the skin and body because it

a) _____

b) _____

c) _____

d) _____

81. Explain how to determine the amount of water needed every day for maximum physical health. _____

_____

82. How many ounces (liters) of water does a person who weighs 175 pounds (79 kg) need to drink each day? _____

83. List six signs that indicate a person is not drinking enough water.

1) _____

2) _____

3) _____

4) _____

5) _____

6) _____

CHAPTER 8 Skin Disorders and Diseases

Date: _____

Rating: _____

Text Pages: 174–195

POINT TO PONDER

"Excellence is not an act, it is a habit."—***Aristotle***

WHY STUDY SKIN DISORDERS AND DISEASES?

1. Skin care is an area of rapid growth in the cosmetology industry.

   _____ True

   _____ False

2. Explain why you think it is important for a beauty professional to be able to recognize different skin disorders and diseases.

   _____

   _____

   _____

   _____

   _____

   _____

   _____

   _____

   _____

   _____

DISORDERS AND DISEASES OF THE SKIN

3. A physician who treats disorders and diseases of the skin is called a(n) _____.

4. A brand new client arrives at your salon for a facial, and you notice she has an inflamed red rash on her chin which she says is "nothing." What should you do?

_____ a) Perform a facial on the client as scheduled, going easy on the chin area.

_____ b) Search online to see if you can identify whether the rash is contagious.

_____ c) Tell her kindly that you cannot perform a facial without a note from her doctor.

5. Explain your answer to question 4: _____

_____

_____

LESIONS OF THE SKIN

6. A(n) _____ is a mark on the skin that could indicate an injury or damage that changes the structure of tissues or organs.

7. The three types of lesions are:

a) _____

b) _____

c) _____

8. Match each of the following primary lesions with its description.

_____ 1. Bulla   a) Spot or discoloration on the skin

_____ 2. Cyst   b) Small blister or sac containing clear fluid; just beneath the epidermis

_____ 3. Macule   c) Swelling

_____ 4. Papule   d) Large blister containing a watery fluid

_____ 5. Pustule   e) Itchy, swollen lesion lasting only a few hours

_____ 6. Tubercle   f) Inflamed pimple containing pus

_____ 7. Tumor   g) Closed, abnormally developed sac, containing fluid, pus, or semifluid

_____ 8. Vesicle   h) Small, circumscribed elevation on the skin containing no fluid

_____ 9. Wheel   i) Abnormal rounded, solid lump within or under the skin

9. A freckle is an example of a:

_____ a) Bulla

_____ b) Macule

_____ c) Papule

_____ d) Tubercle

10. Which of the following primary lesions requires a referral to a physician?

_____ a) Bulla

_____ b) Macule

_____ c) Papule

_____ d) Pustule

11. A(n) _____ lesion is characterized by piles of material on the skin surface or by depressions in the skin surface.

12. Identify the secondary skin lesions as illustrated:

_____   _____

_____   _____   _____

13. Match each of the following secondary lesions with its description.

_____ 1. Crust   a) Skin sore or abrasion produced by scratching or scraping

_____ 2. Excoriation   b) Thick scar resulting from excessive growth of fibrous tissue

_____ 3. Fissure   c) Light-colored, slightly raised mark on the skin formed after injury

_____ 4. Keloid   d) Open lesion on the skin or mucous membrane of
                              the body

_____ 5. Scale   e) Any thin plate of epidermal flakes; dry or oily

_____ 6. Scar   f) Crack in the skin that penetrates the dermis

_____ 7. Ulcer   g) Dead cells that form over a wound or blemish while it
                              is healing

14. Give an example of a scale: _____.

15. Where on the body are fissures most commonly found? _____

_____

16. Another word for scar is _____

17. Which of the seven secondary lesions that were discussed in Chapter 8 of the
textbook require medical referral? _____

DISORDERS OF THE SEBACEOUS (OIL) GLANDS

18. The sebaceous glands of the skin produce _____.

19. Match each of the following disorders of the sebaceous glands with its
description.

_____ 1. Comedo   a) Skin condition caused by inflammation
                                  of the sebaceous glands

_____ 2. Milia   b) Chronic condition appearing primarily
                                  on the cheeks and nose

_____ 3. Acne   c) Hair follicle filled with keratin and sebum

_____ 4. Seborrheic dermatitis   d) Chronic inflammation of the sebaceous
                                      glands caused by bacteria

_____ 5. Rosacea   e) Benign, keratin-filled cysts

20. Comedones may be removed in the salon as long as a cosmetologist has been
trained properly.

_____ True

_____ False

21. What causes sebum to turn black? _____

_____

22. Why does a whitehead not appear black?

_____

_____

DISORDERS OF THE SUDORIFEROUS (SWEAT) GLANDS

23. Match each of following disorders of the sudoriferous glands with its description.

_____ 1. Anhidrosis   a) Foul-smelling perspiration

_____ 2. Bromhidrosis   b) Excessive sweating

_____ 3. Hyperhidrosis   c) Deficiency in perspiration

_____ 4. Miliaria rubra   d) Prickly heat; acute inflammatory disorder of the sweat glands

INFLAMMATIONS AND COMMON INFECTIONS OF THE SKIN

24. Match each of the following skin conditions with its description.

_____ 1. Dermatitis   a) Fever blister or cold sore

_____ 2. Eczema   b) Inflammatory condition of the skin

_____ 3. Herpes simplex   c) Noncontagious skin disease that causes red patches covered with silver-white scales

_____ 4. Psoriasis   d) Inflammatory disease, often accompanied by painful itching

_____ 5. Conjunctivitis   e) Contagious eye infection caused by bacteria

_____ 6. Impetigo   f) Contagious bacterial skin infection that usually appears on the face

25. With treatment, the herpes simplex virus can be completely cured with all traces of the virus removed from the body.

_____ True

_____ False

26. It is possible to get eczema by working on a client who has this condition.

_____ True

_____ False

PIGMENT DISORDERS OF THE SKIN

27. Name six factors that may affect the pigment of the skin.

a) _____

b) _____

c) _____

d) _____

e) _____

f) _____

28. What is the medical term for an abnormal coloration of the skin? _____

29. A darker than normal skin pigmentation is called _____.

30. Light or white splotches on the skin is caused by _____.

31. Match each of the following skin pigmentation disorders with its description.

_____ 1. Albinism   a) Increased pigmentation on the skin

_____ 2. Chloasm   b) Small or large malformation of the skin due to abnormal pigmentation

_____ 3. Lentigines   c) Absence of melanin pigment of the body

_____ 4. Leukoderma   d) Abnormal brown or wine-colored skin discoloration

_____ 5. Nevus   e) Change in pigmentation caused by exposure to the sun or ultraviolet rays

_____ 6. Stain   f) Milky white spots of skin

_____ 7. Tan   g) Skin disorder characterized by light abnormal patches

_____ 8. Vitiligo   h) Technical term for freckles

HYPERTROPHIES OF THE SKIN

32. _____ of the skin is an abnormal growth of the skin.

33. A skin growth that is _____ is harmless.

34. Match the each of the following skin abnormalities with its description.

_____ 1. Keratoma   a) A small, brownish spot or blemish

_____ 2. Mole   b) Technical term for a wart

_____ 3. Skin tag   c) Small brown or flesh-colored outgrowth of the skin

_____ 4. Verruca   d) An acquired, superficial, thickened patch of epidermis

35. A more common name for a keratoma is a(n) _____; a keratoma that grows inward is called a(n) _____.

36. Why can't a trained cosmetologist remove a skin tag for a client?

_____

37. Under what circumstances may a cosmetologist remove a hair from a client's mole?

_____ a) If the client requests it.

_____ b) When the mole is on the client's face.

_____ c) Only if the mole is flat, not rounded.

_____ d) It is never appropriate.

SKIN CANCER

38. What is the main cause of skin cancer? _____

39. _____ is the most common type of skin cancer and is the least severe.

40. _____ is more serious and often is characterized by scaly red papules or nodules.

41. _____ is the most serious form of skin cancer and is often characterized by black or dark brown patches and may appear uneven in texture, jagged, or raised.

42. The least common form of skin cancer is _____.

43. Explain the role of the cosmetologist in detecting skin cancer.

_____

_____

_____

_____

44. List the parts of the ABCDE Cancer Checklist.

A: _____

B: _____

C: _____

D: _____

E: _____

ACNE AND PROBLEM SKIN

45. Acne is considered both a skin _____ and a(n) _____ problem.

46. Acne may occur in a person of any age.

_____ True

_____ False

47. Name the two major factors that cause acne.

a) _____

b) _____

48. What causes the red appearance of pimples? _____

_____

_____

49. Name four basic ways to treat acne.

a) _____

b) _____

_____

c) _____

_____

d) _____

50. A product that is _____ has been designed and proven not to clog the follicles.

51. When is it appropriate for a salon professional to treat a mild or moderate case of acne? _____

AGING SKIN ISSUES

52. Define intrinsic factors that influence skin aging and give three examples.

_____

_____

53. Define extrinsic factors that influence skin aging and give seven examples.

_____

_____

_____

_____

54. Explain why smoking and drinking, when done together, can be damaging to the skin.

_____

_____

_____

55. Discuss at least three damaging effects of illegal drug use on the skin.

_____

_____

_____

56. You are a cosmetologist who lives and works in a large city. What is the best advice you can give clients about performing skin care? _____

_____

_____

_____

_____

57. Damage done by lifestyle changes is hard to reverse or diminish.

_____ True

_____ False

THE SUN AND ITS EFFECTS

58. Approximately 80 to 85 percent of our aging is caused by the _____.

59. As we age, the _____ and _____ of the skin naturally weaken.

60. The ultraviolet rays of the sun reach the skin in two different forms, _____ and _____ rays.

61. UVA rays, also called _____, are deep penetrating rays that weaken the collagen and elastin fibers, causing _____ in the tissues.

62. UVB rays, also referred to as the _____, cause sunburns, tanning, and the majority of skin cancers.

63. List the precautions to take when you will be exposed to the sun.

a) _____

b) _____

c) _____

_____

d) _____

_____

e) _____

f) _____

_____

CONTACT DERMATITIS

64. A skin disorder that is commonly experienced by cosmetologists is

_____.

65. Why are cosmetologists likely to have this condition? _____

_____

_____

66. _____ is an allergic reaction caused by repeated exposure to a chemical or substance.

67. What is the best was to clear up an allergy to a product? _____

_____

_____

68. What are the three most likely places allergies may occur?

a) _____

b) _____

c) _____

69. If the skin is irritated by a substance, it is called _____ contact dermatitis.

70. Name two types of products with irritant potential.

a) _____

b) _____

71. Explain what occurs when the skin is damaged by irritating substances.

_____

_____

72. Describe how cosmetologists can prevent both types of dermatitis while at work.

_____

_____

_____

_____

73. Name three strategies cosmetologists should follow to prevent a skin problem from developing.

a) _____

b) _____

_____

c) _____

Date: _____

Rating: _____

Text Pages: 196–203

POINT TO PONDER:

"He who is afraid of doing too much always does too little."
—German Proverb

1. The _____ is a hard, protective plate located at the end of the finger.

2. Nails are part of what body system? _____

WHY STUDY NAIL STRUCTURE AND GROWTH?

3. A cosmetologist who is unfamiliar with the way natural nails grow will be able to groom, strengthen, and beautify nails expertly.

   _____ True

   _____ False

4. Why do you think it is important for you to understand the growth cycle of the natural nail?

   _____

   _____

   _____

   _____

   _____

THE NATURAL NAIL

5. Another name for the natural nail is the _____.

6. The natural nail is made mostly of a protein called _____.

7. The keratin found in the natural nail is not as hard as the keratin found in the hair or skin.

   _____ a) True

   _____ b) False

8. Describe the appearance of a healthy nail. _____

_____

_____

9. The nail plate is relatively _____ to water, allowing water to pass more easily than it will pass through normal skin of equal thickness.

10. The nail may look dry and hard, but it actually has a water content of between _____ which varies based on the relative humidity of the surrounding environment.

a) 5 and 10 percent

b) 10 and 20 percent

c) 15 and 25 percent

d) 20 and 30 percent

11. Water directly affects the nail's _____; a nail with lower water content is more _____.

12. What can be done to reduce water loss and improve flexibility? _____

_____

NAIL ANATOMY

13. How many main parts is the nail divided into?

_____ a) 5

_____ b) 6

_____ c) 7

_____ d) 8

14. Together, all of the main parts of the nail are referred to as the _____.

15. Identify the parts of the nail as illustrated below:

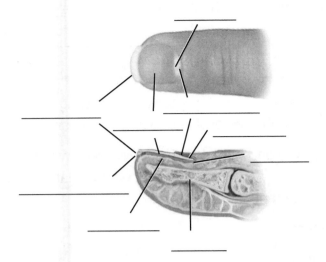

16. The _____ is the most visible and functional part of the nail module. It is constructed of about _____ layers of nail cells.

17. The part of the nail plate that extends over the tip of the finger or toe is the

    _____.

18. Which of the following best describes the nail plate?

    _____ a) Soft

    _____ b) Porous

    _____ c) Dry

    _____ d) Alive

19. The _____ is the portion of living skin on which the nail plate sits.

20. The nail bed is supplied with many nerves and is attached to the nail plate by a thin layer of tissue called the _____.

21. The _____ is where the natural nail is formed.

22. The visible part of the matrix that extends from underneath the living skin is called the _____.

23. Every nail has a lunula.

    _____ True

    _____ False

24. Why is it sometimes difficult to see a lunula? _____

    _____

Courtesy of Godfrey F. Mix, DPM, Sacramento, CA.

25. Name three factors that may affect the growth of the nails.

1) _____

2) _____

3) _____

26. Excessive perspiration from the nail may affect the services a cosmetologist can perform on a client.

_____ True

_____ False

27. The _____ is the dead, colorless tissue attached to the natural nail plate.

28. What is the purpose of the cuticle? _____

_____

_____

29. Which of the following best describes the cuticle?

_____ a) Alive

_____ b) Pigmented

_____ c) Sticky

_____ d) Unimportant

30. The living skin at the base of the nail plate covering the matrix area is the

_____.

31. Describe the difference between the eponychium and the cuticle. _____

_____

_____

32. The _____ is the slightly thickened layer of skin that lies underneath the free edge of the nail plate.

33. What is the function of the hyponychium? _____

_____

_____

34. The cuticle will bleed if it is cut.

_____ True

_____ False

35. Which of the following is easy to remove with gentle scraping?

_____ a) Cuticle

_____ b) Eponychium

36. Which of the following is most likely to need a softener?

_____ a) Cuticle

_____ b) Eponychium

37. A tough band of fibrous tissue that connects bones or holds an organ in place is called a _____.

38. Specialized ligaments attach the nail bed and _____ to the underlying bone and are located at the base of the matrix and around the edges of the nail bed.

39. The _____ are folds of normal skin that surround the nail plate which form nail grooves.

40. The fold of skin that overlaps the side of the nail is called the _____.

41. What are nail grooves? _____

NAIL GROWTH

42. The growth of the nail plate is affected by _____

_____.

43. Describe services a cosmetologist may perform to help make a client's nail plate thicker. _____

_____

44. Explain why toenails are thicker and harder than fingernails. _____

_____

45. Identify the various shapes of nails in the illustration below:

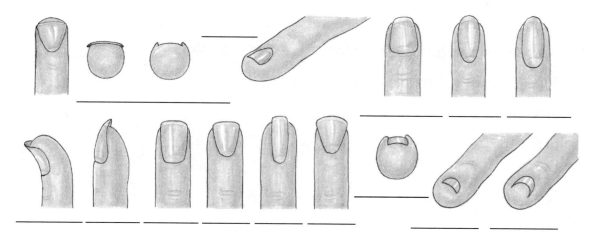

46. The average rate of nail growth in the normal adult is:

_____ a) ½ inch per month.

_____ b) ½ inch per week.

_____ c) ¹⁄₁₀ inch per month.

_____ d) ⅛ inch per week.

47. Nails grow faster in the winter than they do in the summer.

_____ True

_____ False

48. Children's nails grow more rapidly; elderly persons grow at a slower rate.

_____ True

_____ False

49. The nail of the middle finger grows fastest and the thumbnail grows the slowest.

_____ True

_____ False

50. What causes the growth rates of the nail to increase dramatically during

pregnancy? _____

51. A pregnant woman who is taking prenatal vitamins will experience even more rapid nail growth than a pregnant women who is not taking prenatal vitamins.

_____ True

_____ False

52. What will cause the shape or thickness of the nail plate to change? _____

_____

53. How long does replacement of the natural fingernail take? _____

54. Toenails take _____ months to be fully replaced.

    a) 3

    b) 5

    c) 7

    d) 9

55. Like hair, the nail will automatically shed periodically.

    _____ True

    _____ False

KNOW YOUR NAILS

56. A licensed cosmetologist is allowed to:

    _____ Treat nail disorders.

    _____ Clip hangnails upon the client's request.

    _____ Work on healthy nails only.

57. The act of typing helps stimulate nails and make them grow. Why do you think this is the case? Once you have considered your answer, find out if you are correct by searching on-line.

_____

_____

_____

_____

_____

_____

Date: _____

Rating: _____

Text Pages: 204–217

POINT TO PONDER:

"Many things will catch your eye, but only a few will catch your heart...pursue those."—**Unknown**

1. Nails may be described as little _____ that display the overall health of the body.

2. Describe a normal healthy nail. _____

   _____

3. Certain health problems in the body can show up in the nails as visible disorders or poor nail growth.

   _____ True

   _____ False

WHY STUDY NAIL DISORDERS AND DISEASES?

4. It is not the role of the cosmetologist to identify infectious conditions that may be present on a client's nails.

   _____ True

   _____ False

5. Explain why you think it is important for a cosmetologist to be able to recognize nail disorders and diseases when working with clients.

   _____

   _____

   _____

   _____

   _____

   _____

   _____

NAIL DISORDERS

6. A _____ is a condition caused by injury or disease.

7. You can help your clients with nail disorders in what two ways?

   a) _____

   b) _____

   _____

8. When should a client with a nail disorder not receive services? _____
   _____ What should you do if any of these
   are present? _____

9. _____ are a condition in which a blood clot forms under the nail plate,
   forming a dark purplish spot.

10. A noticeably thin, white nail plate that is much more flexible than normal
    is known as a(n) _____; this condition is usually caused by
    _____.

11. Describe the process of manicuring an eggshell nail. _____
    _____
    _____
    _____

12. Visible depressions running across the width of the natural nail plate are
    _____. They usually result from _____ or _____ that has
    traumatized the body.

13. A _____, or agnail, is a condition in which the living skin splits around
    the nail.

14. What will aid in correcting hangnails? _____
    _____

15. Under what circumstances should a cosmetologist intentionally cut or tear a
    client's living skin?

    _____ a) Only when requested to by the client.

    _____ b) Only if the client has an infected hangnail.

    _____ c) Whenever the skin appears to be dry or rough looking.

    _____ d) Under no circumstances.

16. Name four signs of infection: 1) _____, 2) _____, 3) _____,
    4) _____.

17. While working with a client, a cosmetologist may violate a federal regulation as long as a client has given him or her verbal or written permission to do so.

_____ True

_____ False

18. White spots, or _____ spots, are a whitish discoloration of the nails, usually caused by injury to the nail matrix.

19. The darkening of the fingernails or toenails is _____.

20. List three possible causes of discolored nails: 1) _____, 2) _____ , 3) _____.

21. _____, or bitten nails, is the result of a person's habit of chewing the nail or the hardened, damaged skin surrounding the nail plate.

22. The condition of split or brittle nails that also have a series of lengthwise ridges giving a rough appearance to the surface of the nail plate is _____.

23. Onychorrhexis is usually caused by:

a) _____

b) _____

c) _____

d) _____

e) _____

24. It is never appropriate to apply a nail enhancement product if a client's nail bed is exposed.

_____ True

_____ False

25. Plicatured nail literally means _____ and is a type of highly curved nail plate often caused by injury to the _____, but it may be _____.

26. An abnormal condition that occurs when skin is stretched by the nail plate is nail

_____.

27. The terms _cuticle_ and _pterygium_ are the same thing and may be used interchangeably.

_____ True

_____ False

28. Nail pterygium is abnormal damage to the _____ or _____ and should not be treated by pushing the extension of skin back with an instrument.

29. Explain the proper way to care for pterygium. _____

_____

30. _____ run vertically down the length of the natural nail plate and are caused by _____ of the nails, usually the result of _____.

31. What can be done to minimize the appearance of ridges?

a) _____

b) _____

32. Splinter hemorrhages are caused by trauma or injury to the _____.

33. Explain why splinter hemorrhages are always positioned lengthwise in the direction of nail growth. _____

_____

_____

34. Nail plates with a deep or sharp curvature at the free edge have this shape because of the _____; this is known as a _____.

35. _____ are parasites that under some circumstances may cause infections of the feet and hands.

36. Why is nail fungi of concern to a salon? _____

_____

37. Which of the following statements is most accurate?

_____ a) It is highly likely that a client with a nail fungus could infect a cosmetologist.

_____ b) Fungal infections of the fingernail are more common than fungal infections of the toenail.

_____ c) A client with a fungal infection of the toenail could potentially infect another client.

38. How can the transmission of fungal infections be avoided? _____

_____

39. In the past, discolorations of the nail plate were incorrectly referred to as

_____.

40. Nail plate discoloration is usually a _____ infection.

41. Bacterial and fungal organisms both thrive best in dark, moist environments.

_____ True

_____ False

42. Describe the stages of a typical bacterial infection of the nail plate.

_____

_____

43. When is it appropriate for a cosmetologist to treat a client's nail infection?

_____ a) Only if asked by the salon manager.

_____ b) Under no circumstances.

_____ c) If the client is unable to see a physician.

_____ d) In cases where the infection appears mild.

44. Discuss some steps a cosmetologist can take to prevent the transmission of nail infections.

_____

_____

_____

_____

_____

45. When performing a nail enhancement service on a regular client, it is appropriate to skip some disinfection procedures, as long as you know your client does not have a nail infection.

_____ True

_____ False

NAIL DISEASES

46. Are there any nail diseases that should be treated in the salon?

_____ Yes

_____ No

47. Match each of the following nail diseases with its description.

_____ 1. Onychosis   a) Ingrown nails

_____ 2. Onychia   b) The separation and falling off of a nail plate from the nail bed

_____ 3. Onychocryptosis   c) A bacterial inflammation of the tissues surrounding the nail

_____ 4. Onycholysis   d) The medical term for fungal infections of the feet

_____ 5. Onychomadesis e) A severe inflammation of the nail in which a lump of red tissue grows up from the nail bed to the nail plate

_____ 6. Nail psoriasis f) Any deformity or disease of the nail

_____ 7. Paronychia g) The lifting of the nail plate from the bed without shedding

_____ 8. Pyogenic granuloma h) A fungal infection of the nail plate

_____ 9. Tinea pedis i) Tiny pits or severe roughness on the surface of the nail plate

_____ 10. Onychomycosis j) An inflammation of the nail matrix followed by the shedding of the natural nail plate

48. People who work in jobs that require them to place their hands in _____ _____ are more likely to develop nail infections.

49. If you are unsure of how to use a professional product safely, the best way to find out is to:

_____ a) Ask a coworker at the salon.

_____ b) Contact the product manufacturer for the MSDS.

_____ c) Contact the poison control hotline.

_____ d) None of these answers are correct.

50. Which of the following conditions is usually caused by trauma or physical injury?

_____ a) Nail psoriasis

_____ b) Paronychia

_____ c) Onycholysis

_____ d) Onychomycosis

51. A bartender or nurse is most likely to develop which of the following nail infections?

_____ a) Onychomadesis

_____ b) Paronychia

_____ c) Onycholysis

_____ d) Onychocryptosis

11 Properties of the Hair and Scalp

Date: _____

Rating: _____

Text Pages: 218–243

POINT TO PONDER:

"Never give up then, for it is just the place and time that the tide will turn."—**Harriet Beecher Stow**

WHY STUDY PROPERTIES OF THE HAIR AND SCALP?

1. _____ is the scientific study of hair, its diseases, and care, which comes from the Greek words _____, meaning "hair," and _____, meaning "the study of."

2. The hair, skin, and nails are collectively known as the _____.

3. Discuss why you think it is important for you to understand the growth, structure, and composition of hair.

_____

_____

_____

_____

_____

STRUCTURE OF THE HAIR

4. A mature strand of human hair is divided into two parts: the _____, located below the surface of the scalp, and the _____, the portion of the hair that projects above the skin.

5. Match the main structures of the hair root with their description.

_____ 1. Follicle   a) Small, cone-shaped area located at the base of the follicle

_____ 2. Bulb   b) The tube-like depression in the skin or scalp that contains the hair root

_____ 3. Dermal papilla   c) Involuntary muscle in the base of the hair follicle

_____ 4. Arrector pili   d) The oil glands of the skin

_____ 5. Sebaceous glands   e) Thickened, club-shaped structure; forms
                                    the lower part of the root

6. Hair follicles are distributed all over the body, with the exception of:

   a) _____

   b) _____

7. A single hair follicle will only ever produce one hair.

   _____ True

   _____ False

8. The lowest part of the hair strand is called the hair _____.

9. Which part of the root contains the blood and nerve supply that provides the
   nutrients needed for hair growth? _____

10. Which muscle when contracted causes goose bumps? _____

11. The sebaceous glands secrete an oily substance called _____, which
    lubricates the hair and skin.

12. Identify the parts of the skin and hair illustrated below:

13. What are the three main layers of the hair shaft?

    c) _____

    d) _____

    e) _____

14. The outermost layer of the hair is the _____.

15. Describe the cuticle layer. _____

    _____

16. Describe what a healthy cuticle layer protects. _____

_____

17. If you hold a single strand of hair that is still attached to your head and move your fingers down the hair shaft, the hair will feel _____.

18. Why must oxidation haircolors, permanent waving solutions, and chemical hair relaxers have an alkaline pH? _____

_____

19. Which layer of the hair is the cortex? _____

20. What percentage of weight of the hair comes from the cortex?

_____ a) 50 percent

_____ b) 70 percent

_____ c) 80 percent

_____ d) 90 percent

21. Name three different hair properties for which the cortex is responsible.

a) _____

b) _____

c) _____

22. In what layer of the hair do changes involving oxidation haircolor, wet setting, thermal styling, permanent waving, and chemical hair relaxing take place?

_____

23. The _____ is the innermost layer of the hair and is composed of round cells.

24. All hair has three layers.

_____ True

_____ False

25. Identify the cross-section of a hair as illustrated below:

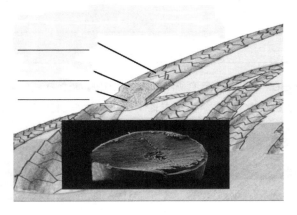

26. How many essential amino acids that are provided only by eating a healthy diet does the body need?

_____ a) 6

_____ b) 9

_____ c) 11

_____ d) 20

27. List some good sources of amino acids.

_____

_____

_____

CHEMICAL COMPOSITION OF HAIR

28. Hair is composed of _____ that grows from cells originating within the hair follicle.

29. The maturation of these cells is a process called _____.

30. Hair is a living thing.

_____ True

_____ False

Explain your answer: _____

_____

31. List the main elements that make up human hair and their percentage in normal hair.

a) _____

b) _____

c) _____

d) _____

e) _____

32. Together, the five elements that make up human hair are known as the _____ elements to help people remember them; they are also found in the _____ and the _____.

33. Match each of the following terms with its description.

_____ 1. Amino acid   a) The chemical bond that links amino acids

_____ 2. Helix   b) The unit of structure that build proteins

_____ 3. Peptide bond   c) A long chain of amino acids linked by peptide bonds

_____ 4. Polypeptide chain   d) The spiral shape of a coiled protein

34. Polypeptide chains are cross-linked together using three different types of side bonds called:

a) _____

b) _____

c) _____

35. A _____ bond is a weak physical side bond that is easily broken by water or heat; these bonds reform when the hair _____.

36. Weak, temporary side bonds between adjacent polypeptide chains are _____ bonds.

37. A _____ bond is a strong chemical side bond that joins the sulfur atom of two neighboring cysteine amino acids to create cystine.

38. How are the hair's strong chemical side bonds broken? _____

_____

_____

39. _____ are the tiny grains of pigment that give natural color to the hair. List and describe the two different types.

a) _____

b) _____

_____

40. How is gray hair different from other hair colors? _____

_____

_____

41. The _____ of the hair refers to the shape of the hair strand and is described as _____ and _____.

42. Natural wave patterns are the result of _____.

43. Asians tend to have _____ hair, while African Americans tend to have _____ hair; however, this is not a hard-and-fast rule and many exceptions exist.

44. In extremely curly hair, cross-sections are usually _____.

45. The shape of a cross-section of hair always relates to the amount of curl in the hair.

_____ True

_____ False

46. Extremely curly hair may have _____ elasticity.

HAIR GROWTH

47. The two main types of hair found on the body are _____ hair and _____ hair.

48. Describe vellus hair. _____
   _____

49. On adults, vellus hair is usually found on the _____
   _____
   _____.

50. Men retain _____ vellus hair than women.

51. Describe terminal hair. _____
   _____

52. Terminal hair is found on the _____
   _____.

53. All hair follicles are able to produce both vellus and terminal hair.

_____ True

_____ False

54. Unscramble these words, then match each word with its correct description.

   gloeten   neanag   agatecn

   _____   The growth phase of new hair

   _____   The transition phase

   _____   The resting phase

55. What is the average growth of healthy scalp hair per month?

_____ a) ¼ inch (0.6 cm)

_____ b) ½ inch (1.25 cm)

_____ c) ¾ inch (1.8 cm)

_____ d) 1 inch (2.5 cm)

56. When does hair tend to grow most rapidly?

_____ a) Between the ages of 8 and 13

_____ b) Between the ages of 15 and 20

_____ c) Between the ages of 15 and 30

_____ d) Between the ages of 40 and 50

57. What percentage of scalp hair is in the catagen phase at any one time?

_____ a) 1 percent

_____ b) 5 percent

_____ c) 10 percent

_____ d) 15 percent

58. What percentage of scalp hair is in the telogen phase at any one time?

_____ a) 1 percent

_____ b) 5 percent

_____ c) 10 percent

_____ d) 15 percent

59. How frequently does the average hair growth cycle take to repeat itself?

_____

60. Shaving, clipping, and cutting the hair makes it grow back faster, darker, and coarser.

_____ True

_____ False

61. Scalp massage increases hair growth.

_____ True

_____ False

62. Gray hair is coarser and more resistant than pigmented hair.

_____ True

_____ False

63. A cross-section of hair can be almost any shape, and its shape does not necessarily relate to the amount of curl in the hair.

_____ True

_____ False

HAIR LOSS

64. It is normal to lose some hair every day.

_____ True

_____ False

65. The average rate of hair loss is _____ hairs per day.

66. Describe why bald and balding men are emotionally affected by their hair loss.

_____

_____

_____

_____

_____

67. While less common than in men, hair loss also affects women.

_____ True

_____ False

68. Abnormal hair loss is called _____.

69. _____, or androgenetic alopecia, is the result of genetics, age, and hormonal changes that cause miniaturization of terminal hair, converting it to _____ hair.

70. In men, androgenic alopecia is known as _____ and usually progresses to the familiar horseshoe-shaped fringe of hair.

71. By the age of 35, what percentage of men and women show some degree of hair loss? _____

72. How many people does androgenic alopecia affect in the United States?

_____ a) Millions

_____ b) Thousands

_____ c) Hundreds

73. What is alopecia areata? _____

_____

_____

74. Alopecia areata that progresses to total scalp hair loss it is called _____
_____. When it results in complete body hair loss, it is called _____
_____.

75. Jane, a client at your salon, gave birth to her first baby three months ago. When
she comes in for a service, she complains that her hair seems to be shedding.
This condition is called _____. You reassure Jane that her hair
growth cycle should eventually return to _____ within about _____.

76. What are the only two products that have been proven to stimulate hair growth
and are approved by the Food and Drug Administration (FDA)? _____
_____.

77. A topical medication that is applied to the scalp twice a day, and is sold over-
the-counter as a nonprescription drug, is _____; the most commonly
known product that contains this drug is called _____.

78. _____ is an oral prescription medication for men only and is more
effective and convenient than its nonprescription counterpart.

79. Why are pregnant women warned against having any contact with the oral
prescription medication used to treat hair loss in men? _____
_____

_____

80. Describe the most common surgical treatment for hair loss.

_____

_____

_____

81. What nonmedical options can a hairstylist offer to counter hair loss?

_____

82. Abnormal hair loss may also be a side effect of _____ or
_____ cancer treatments.

83. Summarize the different possible causes of hair loss.

_____

_____

_____

_____

DISORDERS OF THE HAIR

84. Match each of the following hair disorders with its description.

_____ 1. Canities   a) A condition of abnormal growth of hair

_____ 2. Ringed hair   b) Technical term for gray hair

_____ 3. Hypertrichosis   c) Knotted hair

_____ 4. Trichoptilosis   d) Technical term for beaded hair

_____ 5. Trichorrhexis nodosa   e) Technical term for brittle hair

_____ 6. Monilethrix   f) Characterized by alternating bands of
                                         gray and pigmented hair

_____ 7. Fragilitas crinium   g) Technical term for split ends

85. There are two types of canities. They are _____ and _____
_____.

86. In addition to genetics, _____ and _____ may also cause premature
gray hair.

87. What is an example of hypertrichosis? _____
What are possible treatments? _____

_____

_____

88. Softening the hair with conditioners and moisturizers is often used in the
treatment of _____ and may also help _____, but
will not repair the damage.

DISORDERS OF THE SCALP

89. How many pounds of dead skin does the average person shed each year?

_____

90. What is the difference between dry scalp and dandruff? _____

_____

_____

91. Match each of the following scalp disorders with its definition.

_____ 1. Pityriasis   a) Medical term for ringworm

_____ 2. Tinea   b) Dry, sulfur-yellow, cup-like crusts on the scalp called scutula

_____ 3. Tinea capitis   c) An acute, localized bacterial infection of the hair follicle

_____ 4. Tinea favosa   d) Medical term for dandruff

_____ 5. Scabies   e) An inflammation of the subcutaneous tissue caused by staphylococci

_____ 6. Pediculosis capitis   f) Fungal infection characterized by red papules, or spots at the opening of the hair follicles

_____ 7. Furuncle   g) The infestation of the hair and scalp with head lice

_____ 8. Carbuncle   h) Caused by a parasite called a "mite"

92. Research confirms that dandruff is the result of a fungus called _____, a naturally occurring fungus that is present on all human skin.

93. What is the treatment for dandruff? _____

_____

94. List the two principle types of dandruff and give their characterizations.

a) _____

_____

b) _____

_____

95. What is seborrheic dermatitis? _____

_____

96. Name some causes of dry scalp. _____

_____

_____

97. It is appropriate to perform a service on a client who has a severe case of dandruff.

_____ True

_____ False

98. What does tinea look like? _____

_____

99. Tinea is contagious.

_____ True

_____ False

100. Ringworm is caused by a parasite.

_____ True

_____ False

101. What does tinea barbae affect? _____

_____

102. Which of the following conditions has a distinctive odor?

_____ a) Tinea barbae

_____ b) Scabies

_____ c) Scutula

_____ d) Head lice

103. List the ways head lice are transmitted from an infected person to a noninfected person. _____

_____

104. As a cosmetologist, what are two ways you can help prevent the spread of infectious conditions?

_____

_____

_____

HAIR AND SCALP ANALYSIS

105. What special tools does a cosmetologist need in order to perform a hair analysis?

_____

_____

106. Explain the connection between hair analysis and retailing.

_____

_____

_____

_____

_____

_____

107. List and define the four most important factors to consider in hair analysis.

a) _____

b) _____

c) _____

_____

d) _____

_____

108. What are the classifications of hair texture?

a) _____

b) _____

c) _____

109. All hair on a person's head has the same texture.

_____ True

_____ False

110. Which hair texture has the largest diameter? _____

111. Which hair texture is the most common and is the standard? _____

112. Which hair texture has the smallest diameter and is more fragile? _____

113. Which hair texture usually requires extra processing when applying a product like haircolor? _____

114. Hair density can be classified as:

a) _____

b) _____

c) _____

115. Hair density and hair texture are essentially the same thing.

_____ True

_____ False

116. The average hair density is about _____ hairs per square inch (2.5 square cm), and the average head of hair contains about _____ individual hair strands.

117. Which hair color typically has the lowest density?

_____ a) Brown

_____ b) Blond

_____ c) Red

_____ d) Black

118. The hair's ability to absorb moisture is its _____.

119. The degree of porosity is directly related to _____.
Why? _____

_____

120. A term that means resistant to being penetrated by moisture is _____; a term that means absorbs water easily is _____.

121. Chemical services performed on overly porous hair require

_____.

122. Hair with average porosity is considered _____. Overly porous hair is _____.

123. Hair texture always indicates the hair's porosity; for example, coarse hair always has a low porosity.

_____ True

_____ False

124. Describe how to check porosity. _____

_____

_____

_____

125. In a porosity check, if the hair feels smooth, _____

_____ .

126. In a porosity check, if you can feel a slight roughness, _____

_____ .

127. In a porosity check, if the hair feels very rough or dry or breaks,

_____ .

128. The ability of the hair to stretch and return to its original length without breaking is its _____ .

129. Hair elasticity is an indication of _____

_____ .

130. Wet hair with normal elasticity will stretch up to _____ of its original length and return without breaking. Dry hair stretches about _____ of its length.

131. Which of the following statements is true of hair with low elasticity?

_____ a) Chemical services will require a solution with a higher pH.

_____ b) Hair services should not be performed at all.

_____ c) It may not hold a permanent wave as easily.

132. Hair growth patterns are caused by follicles that grow perpendicular (90-degree angle) to the scalp.

_____ True

_____ False

133. Knowing if a client has a hair growth pattern is an important consideration when helping them select a hairstyle or haircut.

_____ True

_____ False

134. Match each of the following terms with its description.

_____ a) Hair stream   a. Hair following in the same direction

_____ b) Whorl   b. A tuft of hair that stands straight up

_____ c) Cowlick   c. Hair that forms in a circular patter

135. Which of the following is not a cause of dry hair and scalp?

_____ a) Winter weather

_____ b) Desert climate

_____ c) Inactive sebaceous glands

_____ d) Active sebaceous glands

136. Oily hair and scalp is caused by _____ or _____ sebaceous glands and is characterized by a greasy buildup on the scalp and an oily coating on the hair.

137. Dry hair and scalp can be caused by inactive _____ and is aggravated by excessive _____.

138. Oily hair and scalp is characterized by _____

_____.

12 Basics of Chemistry

Date: _____

Rating: _____

Text Pages: 244–261

POINT TO PONDER:

"Success seems to be connected with action. Successful people keep moving. They make mistakes, but they don't quit."—**Conrad Hilton**

WHY STUDY CHEMISTRY?

1. Every product you will use on clients in the salon contains some type of chemical.

   _____ True

   _____ False

2. When you first began studying to become a cosmetologist were you surprised that you would be learning about chemistry? Describe your reaction and why you think it is important for you to learn the basics about chemistry.

   _____

   _____

   _____

   _____

   _____

   _____

   _____

   _____

CHEMISTRY

3. _____ is the science that deals with the composition, structures, and properties of matter and how matter changes under different conditions.

4. _____ is the study of substances that contain carbon.

5. The term organic does not mean "natural."

_____ True

_____ False

6. Anything that is called organic is healthy and safe.

_____ True

_____ False

7. _____ is the study of substances that do not contain carbon.

8. For each of the following substances, write an O if the item is organic and write an I if the item is Inorganic.

_____ Gasoline

_____ Water

_____ Synthetic fabrics

_____ Shampoo

_____ Iron

_____ Air

9. Explain why most inorganic substances do not burn, yet organic substances will burn. _____

_____

_____

_____

_____

MATTER

10. Match each of the following terms with its definition.

_____	1. Matter	a) Simplest form of matter.
_____	2. Elements	b) Chemical combination of two or more atoms.
_____	3. Atoms	c) Any substance that occupies space and has mass.
_____	4. Molecule	d) Particles from which all matter is composed.

11. All matter has physical and chemical properties and exists in the form of a(n) _____, _____, or _____.

12. Everything that is made out of matter is:

_____ a) Organic.

_____ b) Chemical.

_____ c) Inorganic.

13. _____ does not occupy space or have mass.

14. Everything that is known to exist in the universe is made of either _____ or

_____.

15. There are _____ naturally occurring elements, each with its own distinct physical and chemical properties.

16. How are chemical elements identified? _____ Give an example of three elements. _____

17. A(n) _____ is the smallest particle of an element that retains the properties of that element.

18. What makes one element different from another element? _____

_____

19. How are molecules made? _____

20. _____ are a chemical combination of atoms of the same element.

21. _____ are chemical combinations of two or more atoms of different elements.

22. You should use chemical-free products on clients who prefer things that are organic.

_____ True

_____ False

Explain your answer: _____

23. The human body is composed of chemicals.

_____ True

_____ False

24. _____ are the three different physical forms of matter.

25. Match the three different states of matter with their corresponding characteristics.

_____ 1. Solids   a) Do not have a definite shape or volume

_____ 2. Liquids   b) Have a definite shape and volume

_____ 3. Gases   c) Have a definite volume but not a definite shape

26. It is possible for a substance to exist in all _____ forms of matter. Give an example. _____.

27. _____ are those characteristics that can be determined without a chemical reaction and do not include a chemical change. Physical properties include _____.

28. _____ are those characteristics that can only be determined by a chemical reaction and a chemical change in the substance.

29. List two examples of chemical properties. _____

_____

30. A change in the form or physical properties of a substance without a chemical reaction or the creation of a new substance is a(n) _____.

31. What are two examples of a physical change?

a) _____

b) _____

32. A change in the chemical and physical properties of a substance by a chemical reaction is a(n) _____.

33. What is oxidation? _____

_____

34. List two examples of a chemical change.

a) _____

b) _____

35. The contraction *redox* stands for _____ reaction.

36. Explain what happens during redox. _____

_____

_____

37. What is an example of an oxidizing agent? _____

38. What is an example of a reducing agent? _____

_____

39. Define each of the following terms.

a) Oxidizing _____

b) Reducing _____

c) Reduction _____

_____

40. Oxidation and reduction reactions always occur at the same time and are referred to as _____. The reaction involves a transfer between the _____ and the _____.

41. Chemical reactions that produce heat are called _____.

42. All oxidation reactions produce heat.

_____ True

_____ False

43. _____ is the rapid oxidation of substance, accompanied by the production of heat and light.

44. A(n) _____ is a chemical combination of matter in definite proportions.

45. What are some examples of a pure substance? _____

_____

46. A physical mixture is a physical combination of _____ in any proportions.

47. Salt water is an example of a _____.

_____ a) pure substance

_____ b) physical mixture

48. Describe three ways a physical mixture is different from a pure substance.

_____

_____

_____

_____

49. Match each of the following terms with its description.

_____ 1. Solution   a) Stable mixture of two or more mixable substances

_____ 2. Solute   b) The substance that dissolves

_____ 3. Solvent   c) The substance that is dissolved

50. Which of the following is considered the universal solvent?

_____ a) Water

_____ b) Oil

_____ c) Alcohol

51. _____ liquids are mutually soluble, meaning that they can be mixed into stable solutions.

52. _____ liquids are not capable of being mixed into stable solutions.

53. Determine whether each of the following is an example of a miscible (M) liquid, or an immiscible (I) liquid.

_____ a) Water and alcohol.

_____ b) Water and oil.

_____ c) Water and polish remover.

54. An unstable mixture of undissolved particles in a liquid is a(n):

_____ a) Emulsion.

_____ b) Suspension.

_____ c) Surfactant.

55. An unstable mixture of two or more immiscible substances united with the aid of an emulsifier is a(n):

_____ a) Emulsion.

_____ b) Suspension.

_____ c) Surfactant.

56. Substances that act as a bridge to allow oil and water to mix or emulsify are:

_____ a) Emulsions.

_____ b) Suspensions.

_____ c) Surfactants.

57. Give two examples of a suspension.

a) _____

b) _____

58. Which of the following is true about an emulsion?

_____ a) It never separates.

_____ b) It is stable.

_____ c) Nail primer is an example.

_____ d) It separates slowly.

59. A surfactant molecule has two distinct parts. The head is _____, meaning water-loving, and the tail is _____, meaning oil-loving.

60. What does the contraction *surfactant* stand for? _____

61. Why do traditional bar soaps often make people's hands feel itchy after use?

_____

_____

_____

62. An example of an oil-in-water emulsion is _____. Describe why:

_____

_____

63. What are two examples of a water-in-oil emulsion? _____

_____

64. Give four examples of semisolid mixtures that may be used in the salon.

a) _____

b) _____

c) _____

d) _____

65. Isopropyl alcohol and ethyl alcohol are both _____ alcohols.

66. Match each of the following chemical ingredients with its description.

_____ 1. Alkonolamines   a) Special type of oil used in hair conditioners

_____ 2. Ammonia   b) Sweet, colorless, oily substance

_____ 3. Glycerin

c) Substances used to neutralize acids or raise the pH of many hair products

_____ 4. Silicones

d) Contain carbon and evaporate quickly

_____ 5. Volatile organic compounds (VOCs)

e) Colorless gas with a pungent odor

67. The use of this chemical ingredient is not supposed to cause blackheads.

_____ a) Glycerin

_____ b) Silicone

_____ c) Ammonia

_____ d) VOCs

68. These evaporate quickly.

_____ a) Glycerins

_____ b) Silicones

_____ c) Alkonolamines

_____ d) VOCs

POTENTIAL HYDROGEN (pH)

69. What does pH stand for? _____

70. The term _pH_ refers to the quantity of _____.

71. A(n) _____ is an atom or molecule that carries an electrical charge.

72. _____ is the separation of an atom or molecule into positive and negative ions.

73. An ion with a negative electrical charge is an _____; an ion with a positive electrical charge is a _____.

74. Only products that contain water can have a pH.

_____ True

_____ False

75. What does the pH scale measure? _____

76. The pH scale ranges from 0 to 14. Match each of the following pH values with the appropriate solution type.

_____ (b) 1. pH below 7   a) Neutral solution

_____ (a) 2. pH of 7   b) Acidic solution

_____ (c) 3. pH above 7   c) Alkaline solution

77. The term _____ means multiples of 10.

78. A pH of 9 is how many more times more alkaline than a pH of 8?

_____ a) 10 times

_____ b) 100 times

_____ c) 1,000 times

_____ d) None of these answers are true; it is more acidic.

79. Skin and hair have an average pH of _____.

_____ a) 4

_____ b) 5

_____ c) 6

_____ d) 7

80. Explain why pure water alone may be drying to the skin.

_____

_____

_____

81. All _____ owe their chemical reactivity to the hydrogen ion. Acids have a pH below _____.

82. An example of an acid that may be used in the salon is a(n) _____

_____.

83. Acids _____ and _____ the hair.

84. All _____ owe their chemical reactivity to the hydroxide ion. The terms _____ and _____ are interchangeable. Alkalis have a pH above _____.

85. Alkalis _____ and _____ the hair, skin, cuticle, and calloused skin.

86. Another term for sodium hydroxide is _____.

87. Name four safety precautions you should take when working with sodium hydroxide.

a) _____

b) _____

c) _____

d) _____

88. Acids and alkalis, when mixed together in equal proportions, create _____.

89. Neutralizing shampoos and normalizing lotions used to neutralize hydroxide hair relaxers work by creating an acid-alkali _____ reaction.

90. Discuss one way to neutralize alkaline callous softener residues that may be left on a client's skin after rinsing.

_____

13 Basics of Electricity

Date: _____

Rating: _____

Text Pages: 262–280

POINT TO PONDER:

"Success is going from failure to failure without losing your enthusiasm."—**Abraham Lincoln**

WHY STUDY THE BASICS OF ELECTRICITY?

1. As a cosmetologist, you will use many electrical appliances and knowledge of electricity can help you use them safely and effectively. List the electrical appliances you expect to use as cosmetologist. Then, once you have finished reading this chapter in your textbook, recheck your list and add any additional items you did not include the first time.

_____

_____

ELECTRICITY

2. _____ is a form of energy; it is the movement of particles around an atom.

3. When in motion, energy exhibits _____, _____, or _____ effects.

4. A(n) _____ is a flow of electricity along a conductor.

5. Any substance that easily transmits electricity is a _____.

6. Which of the following is a conductor?

_____ a) Wood

_____ b) Copper

_____ c) Cloth

_____ d) Alcohol

7. A substance that does not easily transmit electricity is a(n) _____ or a(n) _____. Name five examples. _____

8. Which of the following is not an insulator?

_____ a) Rubber

_____ b) Silk

_____ c) Cement

_____ d) Water

9. A(n) _____ is the path of negative and positive electric currents from the generating source through the conductor and back to its original source.

10. Static shock is a form of electricity.

_____ True

_____ False

11. Name the two types of electric current.

a) _____

b) _____

12. Direct current is a constant, even-flowing current that travels in _____ direction and is produced by _____.

13. _____ current is a rapid and interrupted current, flowing first in one direction and then in the opposite direction.

14. What apparatus changes direct current to alternating current? _____

15. What apparatus changes alternating current to direct current? _____

16. Name which type of current each of the following items use.

a) Flashlights: _____

b) Curling irons: _____

c) Mobile phones: _____

d) Table lamps: _____

e) Car battery: _____

f) Hot rollers: _____

17. Match each term with its definition.

_____ 1. Volt   a) Measures the strength of an electrical current.

_____ 2. Amp   b) Measures how much electric energy is used in 1 second.

_____ 3. Milliampere   c) Equals 1,000 watts.

_____ 4. Ohm   d) Measures the pressure or force that pushes the
                                flow of electrons through a conductor.

_____ 5. Watt   e) Equals one-thousandth of an ampere.

_____ 6. Kilowatt   f) Measures the resistance of an electric current.

ELECTRICAL EQUIPMENT SAFETY

18. When electrical wires in a wall overheat, the result is a(n) _____.

19. A device that prevents excessive current from passing through a circuit is a

_____.

20. A switch that automatically interrupts or shuts off an electric circuit at the first
indication of overload is a _____.

21. What does UL stand for? _____

22. What does the UL symbol mean when it's found on an electrical appliance?

_____

23. What is grounding? _____

_____

24. List all of the safety guidelines that you should adhere to when using electric
appliances in the salon.

a) _____

b) _____

c) _____

d) _____

e) _____

f) _____

_____

g) _____

_____

h) _____

i) _____

_____

j) _____

k) _____

_____

l) _____

m) _____

_____

n) _____

o) _____

ELECTROTHERAPY

25. _____ are commonly referred to as electrotherapy.

26. A(n) _____ or _____ is an instrument that plugs into an ordinary wall outlet and produces different types of electric currents that are used for _____. They are called _____.

27. A(n) _____, or probe, is an applicator for directing the electric current from the machine to the client's skin and is usually made of _____, _____, or _____ .

28. _____ indicates the negative and positive poles of an electric current. Electrotherapy devices always have one negatively charged pole, called a(n) _____ and one positively charged pole, called a(n) _____.

29. The positive electrode is usually _____ and is marked with a "P" or a plus (+) sign.

30. The negative electrode is usually _____ and is marked with an "N" or minus (–) sign.

31. List the three modalities used in cosmetology.

a) _____

b) _____

c) _____

32. _____ current is constant and direct, with a positive and negative pole, that produces chemical changes when it passes through the tissues and fluids of the body.

33. The electrode used on the area to be treated is the _____ electrode; the _____ electrode is the opposite pole.

34. _____ is the process of infusing water-soluble products into the skin with the use of electric current.

35. _____ forces acidic substances into deeper tissues using galvanic current from the positive toward the negative pole.

36. _____ is the process of forcing liquids into the tissues from the negative toward the positive pole.

37. _____ is a process used to soften and emulsify grease deposits and blackheads in the hair follicles.

38. A client with pustular acne is a good candidate for receiving galvanic current.

_____ True

_____ False

MICROCURRENT

39. An extremely low level of electricity that mirrors the body's natural electrical impulses is called _____.

40. List nine ways this type of low level electricity may be beneficial to clients.

a) _____

b) _____

c) _____

d) _____

e) _____

f) _____

g) _____

h) _____

i) _____

41. The _____ is a thermal or heat-producing current with a high frequency, commonly called the _____ and is used for both scalp and facial treatments.

42. The Tesla current electrodes are made from either _____ or _____.

43. List the benefits from the use of Tesla high-frequency current.

a) _____

b) _____

c) _____

d) _____

e) _____

f) _____

44. Neither Tesla high-frequency current nor microcurrent should be used on female patients who are _____.

OTHER ELECTRICAL EQUIPMENT

45. Give the use or a description of each of the following electrical appliances.

a) Hood hair dryers/heat

lamps   _____

_____

b) Ionic hair dryers   _____

c) Curling and flat irons   _____

_____

d) Heating caps   _____

_____

e) Haircolor processing   _____

machines   _____

_____

f) Steamers or vaporizers   _____

_____

LIGHT ENERGY AND LIGHT THERAPY

46. _____ is electromagnetic radiation that we can see. Electromagnetic radiation is also called _____ because it carries energy through space on waves.

47. The distance between two successive peaks is called the _____.

48. Long wavelengths have low frequency, meaning _____ within a given length. Short wavelengths have higher frequency, meaning _____ within a given length.

49. The _____ is part of the electromagnetic spectrum.

50. Visible light makes up _____ of natural sunlight.

51. _____ and _____ are invisible because their wavelengths are beyond the visible spectrum of light. They make up _____ of natural sunlight.

52. What are some other names for ultraviolet light? _____

_____

53. List six characteristics of ultraviolet light.

a) _____

b) _____

c) _____

d) _____

e) _____

f) _____

g) _____

h) _____

54. Which of the following types of UV light is used in tanning beds?

_____ a) UVA

_____ b) UVB

_____ c) UVC

55. _____ has long wavelengths, penetrates the deepest, and produces the most heat.

56. What are some uses for infrared light in the salon? _____

_____

_____

57. _____ are used to make reactions happen more quickly. They may be either a _____ energy source or a _____ source.

58. What is light therapy? _____

_____

59. What does the acronym laser stand for?

L: _____

A: _____

S: _____

E: _____

R: _____

60. What does the process of selective photothermolysis do?

_____

61. What does LED stand for?

L: _____

E: _____

D: _____

62. Which color LED reduces acne?

_____

63. Which color LED improves collagen and elastin production in the skin?

_____

64. Which color LED reduces inflammation?

_____

65. What is the name of a medical device that is used to treat spider veins, rosacea, and excessive hair?

_____

CHAPTER 14 Principles of Hair Design

Date: _____

Rating: _____

Text Pages: 281–385

POINT TO PONDER:

"A year from now you may wish you had started today."—**Karen Lamb**

WHY STUDY PRINCIPLES OF HAIR DESIGN?

1. When designing a hairstyle for your client, what is your goal?_____

_____

2. A client requests a hairstyle that does not seem to be the right choice for her. Explain why knowing the principles of hair design will help you work with the client to come up with a style that would be more suitable.

_____

_____

_____

_____

_____

_____

PHILOSOPHY OF DESIGN

3. What should a good designer always visualize before beginning?

_____

4. List some sources of inspiration. _____

_____

5. An excellent source of design inspiration may be found in _____.

6. What places, things, or people inspire your creativity? _____

_____

7. In general, hair design usually follows fashion trends.

_____True

_____False

8. Once you have been inspired, what is the next step? _____

_____

9. You have been inspired by a painting and want to try out a new design. Where should you begin?

_____ a) On your next client

_____ b) On yourself

_____ c) On a mannequin head

10. As a designer, what must you develop? _____

_____

11. Understanding which hairstyles work best cannot be achieved through book learning; the best teacher is _____

_____.

12. Having a strong foundation in techniques and skills will allow you to take

_____.

13. A stylist who gives the same haircut to every client is known as a(n):

_____ a) Risk-taker.

_____ b) Outside-the-box innovator.

_____ c) Cookie-cutter designer.

14. What does it mean to "think outside of the box"? _____

_____

_____

_____

_____

ELEMENTS OF HAIR DESIGN

15. What are the five basic elements of three-dimensional design?

a) _____

b) _____

c) _____

d) _____

e) _____

16. _____ create the shape, design, and movement of a hairstyle. They can be _____ or _____ .

17. Match each of the four basic types of lines with its description.

_____ 1. Horizontal lines   a) Lines are up and down

_____ 2. Vertical lines   b) Large or small, a full circle or just part of a circle

_____ 3. Diagonal lines   c) Positioned between horizontal and vertical lines

_____ 4. Curved lines   d) Extend in the same direction and maintain a constant distance apart

18. Describe the usage of the basic types of lines.

a) Horizontal lines: _____

b) Vertical lines: _____

c) Diagonal lines: _____

_____

d) Curved lines: _____

19. A client would like a hairstyle that minimizes her large nose. Which type of line might be most helpful in a design to meet this goal? _____

20. Describe a single line in hairstyling. _____

_____

21. Describe a parallel line in hairstyling. _____

_____

22. Describe a contrasting line in hairstyling. _____

_____

_____

23. Describe a transitional line in hairstyling. _____

_____

24. Describe a directional line in hairstyling. _____

_____

25. _____ is a mass or general outline of a hairstyle that is three-dimensional and has _____, _____, and _____.

26. Another word for form or mass is _____.

27. The _____ is usually the part of the overall design that a client will respond to first.

28. The hair form should be in proportion to the:

a) _____

b) _____

c) _____

29. _____ is the area surrounding the form or the area the hairstyle occupies and may contain _____, _____, _____, _____, or any combination.

30. People usually pay more attention to _____ spaces.

_____ Positive

_____ Negative

31. Wave patterns or _____ must be considered when designing a style for a client.

32. All hair has a natural wave pattern described as:

a) _____

b) _____

c) _____

d) _____

33. Choose one (or more) of the natural wave patterns you just identified in Question 32 to complete the following.

a) These types of wave patterns may be. coarse to the touch:

_____.

b) This type of wave pattern reflects the most light: _____.

c) You can create horizontal lines with this type of wave pattern: _____.

34. How can texture be created temporarily? _____

_____

35. List 10 techniques or tools that will temporarily change hair texture.

a) _____   f) _____

b) _____   g) _____

c) _____   h) _____

d) _____   i) _____

e) _____   j) _____

36. How can texture be changed permanently? _____

37. How long does a permanent texture change last? _____

_____

38. When is it appropriate to use many wave pattern combinations together?

_____

_____

39. _____ wave patterns accent the face and are useful when you wish to narrow a round head shape.

40. _____ wave patterns take attention away from the face and can be used to soften square or rectangular features.

41. What two roles does color play in hair design?

a) _____

b) _____

42. Discuss why you think that hair color is important to the client psychologically in the overall look of a hair design.

_____

_____

_____

_____

_____

_____

43. _____ can be used to make all or part of the design appear larger or smaller and can help define _____ and _____.

44. Light colors and warm colors create the illusion of _____.

45. _____ and _____ colors recede or move in toward the head, creating the illusion of less volume.

46. Explain how to create the illusion of dimension or depth. _____

_____

_____

47. Using a(n) _____ color will draw a line in the hairstyle in the direction you want the eye to travel.

48. How might you use color to create a dramatic accent? _____

_____

49. What should be considered when choosing a color? _____

_____

50. A client with a gold skin tone would look best with a _____ haircolor.

_____ Cool

_____ Warm

51. High contrast colors work best for a conservative look.

_____ True

_____ False

PRINCIPLES OF HAIR DESIGN

52. The five principles for art and design of hair design are:

a) _____

b) _____

c) _____

d) _____

e) _____

53. Match each of the following principles of design with its description.

_____ 1. Proportion   a) Where the eye is drawn to first

_____ 2. Balance   b) Creation of unity

_____ 3. Rhythm   c) Establishing equal or appropriate proportions to create symmetry

_____ 4. Emphasis   d) Regular pulsation or recurrent pattern of movement in a design

_____ 5. Harmony   e) Comparative relationship of one thing to another

54. When designing a hairstyle it is essential that you take into account the client's

_____.

55. What style would you normally create for a woman with large hips or broad shoulders?_____

Explain your answer:_____

56. What is the general guide for "classic" proportion?_____

_____

57. Which element of design can be either symmetrical or asymmetrical?_____

58. Explain how to measure symmetry._____

_____

_____

59. Describe symmetrical balance. _____

_____

_____

_____

60. Describe asymmetrical balance. _____

_____

_____

_____

61. Define _rhythm_ in a design. _____

_____

62. Which of the following signifies a fast rhythm?

_____ a) Tight curls

_____ b) Loose curls

63. What is meant by emphasis in a design?

_____

64. List four options you may choose to create interest in a hairstyle.

a) _____

b) _____

c) _____

d) _____

65. A hair design should have only one point or area of emphasis.

_____ True

_____ False

66. Explain the importance of harmony in a hair design.

_____

67. Name three elements that will make a hairstyle harmonious.

a) _____

b) _____

c) _____

68. A successful harmonious design has an area of emphasis.

_____ True

_____ False

69. The best results are obtained when your client's facial features are properly analyzed for their _____ and _____.

70. An artistic and suitable hairstyle will take into account the following characteristics of the client:

a) _____

b) _____

c) _____

INFLUENCE OF HAIR TYPE ON HAIRSTYLE

71. Hair type is a major consideration in the selection of a hairstyle. What are the two main characterizations to consider?_____

72. List the three main types of hair texture.

1) _____

2) _____

3) _____

73. Match each of the following hair textures with its description.

_____ 1. Fine, straight hair	a) Offers the most versatility in styling
_____ 2. Straight, medium hair	b) Hard to curl; responds well to thermal styling
3. Straight, coarse hair _____	c) Often separates, revealing the client's scalp
_____ 4. Wavy, fine hair	d) Generally best left short
_____ 5. Wavy, medium hair	e) When left natural gives a soft romantic look
_____ 6. Wavy, coarse hair	f) Can get very wide, rather than longer, as it grows
_____ 7. Curly, fine hair	g) Hugs the head shape because of no body or volume
_____ 8. Curly, medium hair	h) May appear fuller with appropriate haircut and style; hair can be fragile
_____ 9. Curly, coarse hair	i) Will be extremely wide without proper maintenance
_____ 10. Very curly, fine hair	j) Needs heavy styling products to weight it down
_____ 11. Extremely curly, medium hair	k) Hair could appear unruly if it is not shaped properly
_____ 12. Extremely curly,	l) Offers more versatility; good amount of coarse hair movement

CREATING HARMONY BETWEEN HAIRSTYLE AND FACIAL STRUCTURE

74. A client's facial shape is determined by the _____ and _____ of the facial bones.

75. What is the best way to determine a client's facial shape?

_____

_____

76. List the seven basic facial shapes.

a) _____

b) _____

c) _____

d) _____

e) _____

f) _____

g) _____

77. When designing a style for your client's facial type, you generally are trying to create the illusion of an _____ -shaped face.

78. To determine a facial shape, divide the face into _____ zones. They are

_____

79. Describe the facial contour of the oval face. _____

_____

_____

80. What type of hairstyle works best on a client with an oval face? _____

_____

_____

81. Describe the facial contour, the aim, and the styling choice for the round-shaped face.

Contour: _____

Aim: _____

Styling choice: _____

_____

82. Describe the facial contour, the aim, and the styling choice for the square-shaped face.

Contour: _____

_____

Aim: _____

Styling choice: _____

_____

83. Describe the facial contour, the aim, and the styling choice for the triangular-shaped (pear-shaped) face.

Contour: _____

Aim: _____

Styling choice: _____

84. Describe the facial contour, the aim, and the styling choice for the oblong-shaped face.

Contour: _____

Aim: _____

Styling choice: _____

_____

85. Describe the facial contour, the aim, and the styling choice for the diamond-shaped face.

Contour: _____

_____

Aim: _____

Styling choice: _____

_____

86. Describe the facial contour, the aim, and the styling choice for the inverted triangle-shaped (heart-shaped) face.

Contour: _____

Aim: _____

_____

Styling choice: _____

_____

87. A long hairstyle is not usually recommended for a client with a(n) _____ facial type.

_____ a) Inverted triangle

_____ b) Square

_____ c) Oblong

_____ d) Oval

88. Bangs are often recommended in hairstyles for clients who have a(n) _____ facial type.

_____ a) Inverted triangle

_____ b) Square

_____ c) Oblong

_____ d) Oval

89. The _____ is the outline of the face, head, or figure seen in a side view.

90. Match each of the following basic profiles with its description.

_____ 1. Straight   a) Has a prominent forehead and chin

_____ 2. Convex   b) Considered ideal; has slight curvature

_____ 3. Concave   c) Has receding forehead and chin

91. This profile type looks best with hairstyles that includes bangs or curls over the forehead. _____

92. This profile type looks best when the hair at the nape of the neck is styled softly upward. _____

93. How should you style the hair for a wide forehead? _____

_____

94. How should you style the hair for a narrow forehead? _____

_____

95. A large forehead looks best with bangs that have a large amount of volume.

_____ True

_____ False

96. How should you style the hair for close-set eyes? _____

_____

_____

97. A subtle lightening of the hair at the corner of the eyes is recommended for wide-set eyes.

_____ True

_____ False

98. How should you style the hair for wide-set eyes? _____

_____

99. How should you style the hair for a crooked nose? _____

_____

100. How should you style the hair for a wide, flat nose?_____

_____

101. How should you style the hair for a long, narrow nose?

_____

_____

102. A hairstyle with a middle part is not recommended for a client who has a long, narrow nose.

_____ True

_____ False

103. Provide the correct styling tip for the following facial features.

a) Round jaw: _____

b) Square jaw: _____

c) Long jaw: _____

_____

d) Receding forehead: _____

_____

e) Large forehead: _____

f) Small nose: _____

g) Prominent nose: _____

_____

h) Receding chin: _____

i) Small chin: _____

j) Large chin: _____

104. How should you style the hair for a head that is not completely round? _____

_____

_____

105. What is a major consideration when creating a hairstyle for someone who wears glasses? _____

_____

106. Where is the bang or fringe area located? _____

_____

107. List the three ways that the bang area or fringe can be parted.

a) _____

b) _____

c) _____

108. List the four parts that can be used to highlight facial features.

a) _____   c) _____

b) _____   d) _____

109. Choose the correct part type from the list above to complete the following.

a) This can help make thinning hair look fuller: _____.

b) This should not be used on a client who has a large nose: _____.

c) This is used to create a dramatic effect: _____.

d) This can help create an illusion of width: _____.

DESIGNING FOR MEN

110. As a professional, what type of styles should you recommend? _____

_____

111. Men are limited by few hairstyle options.

_____ True

_____ False

112. Mustaches and beards can be a great way to _____ on male clients.

113. A man who is balding with closely trimmed hair could also look very good in a closely groomed _____

15 Scalp Care, Shampooing, and Conditioning

Date: _____

Rating: _____

Text Pages: 306–341

POINT TO PONDER

"Formula for Success: Instruction + Example (X) Experience = Success"—**Unknown**

1. One of the most important experiences that a stylist provides is the _____ which can be heavenly, forgettable, or even a nightmare.

2. The "shampoo" actually consists of the following three parts: _____ _____, _____, and _____.

3. Shampooing is an important preliminary step that prepares the hair for a variety of services; it can also be:

   a) _____

   b) _____

WHY STUDY SCALP CARE, SHAMPOOING AND CONDITIONING?

4. The impression you make on a client during the shampoo helps set the tone for the entire service. Explain what you think this means.

   _____

   _____

   _____

   _____

   _____

   _____

5. As long as clients look great when they leave the salon, how they handle their home-care regimen is unimportant to you as a professional.

   _____ True

   _____ False

Explain your answer: _____

_____

_____

_____

SCALP CARE AND MASSAGE

6. List the two basic requirements for a healthy scalp.

   1) _____

   2) _____

7. You should not perform a scalp massage on a scalp that has abrasions.

   _____ True

   _____ False

8. During a service, when is a scalp massage performed on a client?

   1) _____

   2) _____

9. The same products are used for both relaxation and treatment massages.

   _____ True

   _____ False

10. Explain what the term *contraindicated* means in relation to scalp massage.

    _____

    _____

    _____

    _____

11. A client who has high blood pressure should never have a scalp massage.

    _____ True

    _____ False

    Explain your answer: _____

    _____

    _____

    _____

12. If you are unsure about whether it would appropriate to perform a scalp massage on a client who has a medical condition, the best course would be to:

_____ a) Avoid performing the massage.

_____ b) Assume it is fine since the client does not have a doctor's note.

_____ c) Skip the shampoo service.

13. List the four different types of scalp treatments.

a) _____

b) _____

c) _____

d) _____

14. Complete the following by listing the appropriate type of scalp treatment.

a) This may be done in combination with a scalp steamer: _____

_____

b) The main goal of this treatment is to maintain the scalp and hair in a clean and healthy condition: _____

c) A client may need to have this treatment many times: _____

d) This treatment is performed for clients who have overactive sebaceous glands: _____

15. Dandruff is caused by a(n) _____ that is called _____.

BRUSHING THE HAIR

16. List three benefits of correct hair brushing.

a) _____

b) _____

c) _____

17. Do not brush a client's hair if it is oily.

_____ True

_____ False

18. Name two times you should avoid brushing a client's hair.

a) _____

b) _____

19. You should you not brush, massage, or shampoo a client before performing which four services?

a) _____

b) _____

c) _____

d) _____

20. The best type of hairbrush to use for brushing hair is one that has _____ bristles.

_____ a) Natural

_____ b) Plastic

_____ c) Nylon

UNDERSTANDING SHAMPOO

21. The shampoo provides a good opportunity to _____ the client's hair and scalp.

22. What conditions should you check for during the shampoo?

a) _____

b) _____

c) _____

d) _____

e) _____

f) _____

g) _____

h) _____

i) _____

23. A client appears to have a scalp disease that may be infectious. What should you do?

_____

_____

24. The primary purpose of a shampoo is to _____ the hair and scalp prior to a service.

25. To be effective, a shampoo must _____

_____.

26. You should advise all clients to wash their hair every day.

_____ True

_____ False

27. What does excessive shampooing do? _____

_____

28. Oily hair should be shampooed more often than normal or dry hair.

_____ True

_____ False

29. Describe two ways you can help protect yourself from muscle strain and other physical problems that may be caused by performing shampoos on clients.

a) _____

_____

b) _____

30. Professional cosmetologists take time to read product _____ because doing this will help them make informed decisions about what products will work best on individual clients.

31. How should you select a shampoo for a client? _____

_____

32. Hair can usually be characterized as:

a) _____

b) _____

c) _____

d) _____

33. Hair is not considered normal or virgin if it has been _____.

34. List four examples of ways hair may be chemically treated.

a) _____

b) _____

c) _____

d) _____

35. List three ways hair may be damaged.

a) _____

b) _____

c) _____

36. Discuss why it is important to educate clients about which products they should be using for home care.

_____

_____

_____

_____

37. The amount of _____ in a solution is what determines whether it is alkaline or acid.

38. A pH scale ranges from:

_____ a) 0–8

_____ b) 0–12

_____ c) 0–14

_____ d) 0–18

39. A neutral shampoo has a pH of ____.

40. A shampoo that is more _____ can have a pH ranging from 0 to 6.9.

41. A shampoo that is more _____ can have a pH rating of 7.1 or higher.

42. The _____ the pH rating, the stronger and harsher the shampoo.

43. A slightly _____ shampoo more closely matches the ideal pH of hair.

44. When giving a shampoo, you determine if the temperature of the water is comfortable.

_____ True

_____ False

45. Why should you avoid touching a female client's face with your hands, the towel, or water while performing a shampoo? _____

_____

46. It is easy to miss which of the following when performing a shampoo?

_____ a) The bang area

_____ b) Behind the ears

_____ c) The top of the head

_____ d) The nape of the neck

47. Water is classified as a(n) _____ because it is capable of dissolving more substances than any other solvent known to science.

48. Water that comes from a public water system often has _____ added to it to kill _____.

49. The process of heating water to make it a vapor, and then condensing the purified vapor so that it collects as a liquid is called _____.

50. _____ is rainwater or chemically treated water.

51. _____ is often in well-water and contains certain minerals that lessen the ability of soap or shampoo to lather readily.

52. Why is it important for you to understand the classification of the water in the salon where you work? _____

_____

53. Water is the main ingredient in most shampoos.

_____ True

_____ False

54. What is deionized water? _____

_____

_____

55. Surfactant and detergent mean the same thing: _____

_____.

56. A surfactant molecule has two ends: a _____ or water-attracting "head," and a _____ or oil-attracting "tail."

57. During the shampoo process, the hydrophilic head attracts _____ and the lipophilic tail attracts _____.

58. What does the process create? _____

_____

_____

59. List six ingredients that may be added to base surfactants to create a shampoo.

a. _____	d. _____
b. _____	e. _____
c. _____	f. _____

60. Match each type of shampoo with its purpose.

_____ 1. Acid-balanced shampoos	a) Contain special chemicals or drugs to reduce dandruff
_____ 2. Conditioning shampoos	b) Wash away excess oiliness, while keeping the hair from drying out
_____ 3. Medicated shampoos	c) Designed to make the hair smooth and shiny
_____ 4. Clarifying shampoos	d) Used to brighten, add slight color, eliminate unwanted tones
_____ 5. Balancing shampoos	e) Special solutions available for hair enhancements
_____ 6. Dry or powder shampoos	f) Balanced to the pH of skin and hair
_____ 7. Color-enhancing shampoos	g) Cleanse the hair without the use of soap and water
_____ 8. Shampoos for hairpieces/wigs	h) Cut through product buildup
_____ 9. Conditioning shampoos	i) Recommended for color-treated or lightened hair
_____ 10. pH-balanced shampoos	j) Will not strip artificial color from hair

61. How should you shampoo a client who is in a wheelchair?

_____

_____

_____

UNDERSTANDING CONDITIONERS

62. _____ are special chemical agents applied to the hair to deposit protein or moisturizer, to help restore its strength and give it body, or to protect it against possible breakage.

63. Conditioners can heal damaged hair and can improve the quality of new hair growth.

    _____ True

    _____ False

64. What are the three basic types of conditioners?

    a) _____

    b) _____

    c) _____

65. What are humectants? _____

    _____

66. Why is silicone often added to conditioners? _____

    _____

67. Explain what conditioners do: _____

    _____

68. The cortex accounts for what percentage of the hair strand?

    _____ a) 25%

    _____ b) 60%

    _____ c) 75%

    _____ d) 90%

69. _____ are designed to penetrate the cortex and reinforce the hair shaft from within, temporarily reconstructing the hair.

70. The shampoo is a good time for the cosmetologist to:

    _____ a) Educate clients about products

    _____ b) Catch up on news

    _____ c) Relax

    _____ d) All of these answers are correct.

71. List and describe four additional conditioning agents to be familiar with.

   a) _____

   _____

   b) _____

   c) _____

   d) _____

72. A client who has coarse and extremely curly hair would benefit most from which of the following products?

   _____ a) Light leave-in conditioner

   _____ b) Protein and moisturizing treatment

   _____ c) Spray-on thermal protection

   _____ d) pH/acid balanced shampoo

73. A client who has straight, fine hair would benefit most from which of the following products?

   _____ a) Leave-in conditioner

   _____ b) Protein

   _____ c) Finishing rinse

   _____ d) Volumizing shampoo

74. _____, also known as hair masks or conditioning packs, are chemical mixtures of concentrated protein in a heavy base of moisturizer.

DRAPING

75. List the two types of draping that are used on clients.

   a) _____

   b) _____

76. How many times should a client who is having both a shampoo and a chemical service be draped?

   _____ a) Once only

   _____ b) Twice

   _____ c) At least three times

77. Describe why you think it is important for you to learn how to drape a client properly.

_____

_____

_____

_____

_____

_____

_____

20 Chemical Texture Services

Date: _____

Rating: _____

Text Pages: 562–625

POINT TO PONDER:

"Don't confuse fame with success. Madonna is one; Helen Keller is the other."—**Erma Bombeck**

WHY STUDY CHEMICAL TEXTURE SERVICES?

1. Stylists and clients think of chemical texture services as _____ solvers.

2. Why do you think a stylist who performs chemical texture services should have a basic understanding of chemistry?

_____

_____

_____

_____

3. _____ services permanently alter the natural wave pattern of the hair.

4. Texture services can be used to add _____ to straight hair, _____ overly curly hair, or _____ coarse hair to make it more pliable and easier to work with.

5. Chemical textures services include:

   a) _____

   b) _____

   c) _____

THE STRUCTURE OF HAIR

6. The _____ layer is the tough exterior layer of the hair. It surrounds the inner layers and _____ the hair from damage.

7. The cuticle is not directly involved in the texture or movement of the hair.

_____ True

_____ False

8. The _____ is the middle layer of the hair. It is responsible for the _____ and _____ of the human hair.

9. To change the hair's natural wave pattern, it is necessary to _____ the side bonds of the _____.

10. The _____ is often called the pith or core of the hair and does not play a role in structuring or restructuring the hair.

11. Fine hair may not contain which of the following parts?

_____ a) Cuticle

_____ b) Cortex

_____ c) Medulla

12. What does the term pH mean? _____

13. What does the pH scale measure? _____

14. What is the natural pH of hair? _____

15. An acidic substance has a pH of _____.

16. An alkaline substance has a pH of _____.

17. Explain what chemical texturizers do to change the hair's natural curl pattern.

_____

_____

_____

18. Coarse, resistant hair with a strong, compact cuticle layer requires a highly alkaline chemical solution.

_____ True

_____ False

19. Match each term with its definition.

_____ 1. Amino acids	a) Formed by peptide bonds that are linked together.
_____ 2. Peptide bonds	b) Cross-linked polypeptide chains.
_____ 3. Polypeptide chains	c) Compounds made up of carbon, oxygen, hydrogen, and nitrogen.

_____ 4. Keratin proteins	d) Weak physical side bonds that are the result of an attraction between opposite electrical charges.
_____ 5. Side bonds	e) Weak physical side bonds that are the result of an attraction between negative and positive electrical charges.
_____ 6. Disulfide bonds	f) Chemical side bonds that are formed when two sulfur type chains are joined together.
_____ 7. Salt bonds	g) Long, coiled polypeptide chains.
_____ 8. Hydrogen bonds	h) End bonds; link amino acids together in long chains.

20. How are salt bonds broken? _____

21. Hair has the least amount of which type of bonds? _____

PERMANENT WAVING

22. What are the two steps of the permanent wave process?

a) _____

b) _____

_____

23. It is important to do an elasticity test before perming hair.

_____ True

_____ False

24. In permanent waving, the size of the rod determines the _____.

25. _____ are the most common type of perm rod. They have a smaller _____ in the center that increases to a larger circumference on the ends.

26. Concave rods produce a _____ in the center and a _____ on either side of the strand.

27. _____ are equal in diameter along their entire length or curling area.

28. Straight rods produce a _____ along the entire width of the strand.

29. _____ are usually about 12-inches (30.5 cm) long with a uniform diameter along the entire length.

30. What allows these soft foam roads to bend into almost any shape? _____

_____

31. The _____ or _____ rod is usually about 12-inches (30.5 cm) long with a uniform diameter along the entire length of the rod.

32. What does perming only the base of the hair achieve? _____

_____

33. _____ are absorbent papers used to control the ends of the hair when wrapping and winding hair on the perm rods.

34. End papers are also called _____.

35. Why is important to extend end papers beyond the ends of the hair?

_____

36. List the three most common end paper techniques and explain each.

a) _____

_____

b) _____

_____

c) _____

_____

37. All perm wraps begin by sectioning the hair into _____.

38. How do you determine the size, shape, and direction of panels? _____

_____

39. Each panel is divided into subsections called _____.

40. _____ refers to the position of the rod in relation to its base section, and it is determined by the angle at which the hair is wrapped.

41. In what three ways can rods be wrapped?

a) _____

b) _____

c) _____

42. It is common practice to use a base section that is wider than the perm rod.

_____ True

_____ False

43. For on-base placement, the hair is wrapped _____ beyond perpendicular to its base section.

44. Half off-base placement refers to wrapping the hair at a _____ angle or straight out from the center of the section.

45. Half off-base placement _____ stress and tension on the hair.

46. Off-base placement refers to wrapping the hair at _____ below the center of the base section.

47. Which placement creates the least amount of volume and results in curl patterns that begin farthest away from the scalp? _____

48. Base direction refers to the angle at which the rod is positioned on the head _____, _____, or _____.

49. Why is it important to remember to wrap in the natural direction of hair growth?
_____

50. What are the two methods of wrapping the hair around the perm rod?

a) _____

b) _____

51. In which wrapping method is the hair strand wound around the rod, going from the ends to the scalp? _____

52. Which wrapping method produces a uniform curl from the scalp to ends?
_____

53. Which wrapping method produces tighter curl at the ends, and a larger curl at the scalp? _____

54. What is a double-rod or piggyback wrap, and when is it beneficial?

_____

_____

_____

55. What is the benefit of wrapping long hair in a piggyback wrap? _____

_____

56. What does an alkaline permanent waving solution do? _____

_____

57. Once the waving solution is in the cortex, what occurs? _____

_____

58. What is a reduction reaction? _____

_____

59. What is a reduction reaction in permanent waving? _____

_____

60. Explain the chemical process of permanent waving.

1) _____

2) _____

_____

3) _____

_____

4) _____

_____

61. What is the reducing agent used in permanent waving solutions? _____

_____

62. _____ is the most common reducing agent.

63. The strength of the permanent waving solution is determined by _____

_____.

64. Why is ammonia added to the thioglycolic acid product? _____

_____

_____

65. The new chemical created is called _____ and is
the active ingredient or reducing agent in alkaline permanents.

66. Which type of hair will need a more alkaline solution to achieve permanent
waving? _____

67. The first _____ were developed in 1941 and relied on the same ATG
that is still used today.

68. Another name for them is _____.

69. Most alkaline waves have a pH between _____.

70. _____ is an acid with a low pH and is the primary
reducing agent in all modern acid waves.

71. The first _____ were introduced in the early 1970s and have a pH
between _____. They require _____ to speed up processing.

72. What are the three separate components of all acid waves?

a) _____

b) _____

c) _____

73. Most acid waves today have a pH between:

_____ a) 5.8 and 6.2

_____ b) 6.8 and 7.2

_____ c) 7.8 and 8.2

_____ d) 8.8 and 9.2

74. _____ process more quickly and produce firmer curls than true acid waves.

75. _____ create an exothermic chemical reaction that heats up the solution and speeds up the processing.

76. What are the three components of exothermic waves?

a) _____

b) _____

c) _____

77. Mixing an oxidizer with permanent waving solution causes _____

_____

_____.

78. _____ are activated by an outside heat source, usually a conventional hood-type dryer.

79. _____ use an ingredient that does not evaporate as readily as ammonia, so there is very little odor associated with their use.

80. Ammonia-free waves will not damage hair, even if used incorrectly.

_____ True

_____ False

81. Where can you find information about the chemicals contained in a permanent wave product? _____

_____

82. _____ use an ingredient other than ATG as the primary reducing agent.

83. The use of sulfates, sulfites, and bisulfites present an alternative to ATG known as _____.

84. Sulfite permanents are mainly used for _____.

85. The strength of any permanent wave is based on the concentration of its _____.

86. The amount of processing during a permanent wave is determined by the _____ of the permanent waving solution.

87. In permanent waving, most of the processing takes place as soon as the solution _____, within the first 5 to 10 minutes.

88. What does the additional processing time allow? _____

_____

89. When does overprocessing usually occur? _____

90. Resistant hair may not become completely saturated with just one application of waving solution.

_____ True

_____ False

91. To achieve curlier hair, always process it longer.

_____ True

_____ False

92. What occurs if the hair is underprocessed? _____

_____

93. _____ is the process that stops the action of a permanent waving solution and rebuilds the hair into its new form.

94. What are the two important functions of neutralization?

a) _____

b) _____

95. The most common neutralizer is _____.

96. When rinsing perm solution from hair, how long should you rinse? _____

_____

97. If the hair is insufficiently blotted, what will occur? _____

_____

98. Oxidative reactions can _____ hair color, especially at an alkaline pH.

99. When rinsing the hair, you should always use hot water.

_____ True

_____ False

100. When rinsing the hair, use a gentle stream of water.

_____ True

_____ False

101. How should you towel-blot the hair after rinsing? _____

_____

102. Always adjust any rods that have become _____ prior to applying the neutralizer.

103. After rinsing, you should be able to _____ any perm solution that has been left in the hair.

104. _____ breaks disulfide bonds by adding hydrogen atoms to the sulfur atoms. _____ rebuilds the disulfide bonds by removing the extra hydrogen atoms.

105. What information do you obtain from preliminary test curls?

a) _____

b) _____

c) _____

106. List six basic wrapping patterns that are used in permanent waving.

a) _____

b) _____

c) _____

d) _____

e) _____

f) _____

107. Your client would like more volume in one specific area. A solution might be to use a(n) _____.

108. Permanent waving a man's hair requires the use of different techniques than perming a woman's hair.

_____ True

_____ False

109. List the safety precautions for permanent waving.

a) _____

b) _____

_____

c) _____

_____

d) _____

e) _____

_____

f) _____

g) _____

h) _____

i) _____

j) _____

k) _____

l) _____

CHEMICAL HAIR RELAXERS

110. _____ is the process of rearranging the basic structure of extremely curly hair into a straighter or smoother form.

111. The chemistry of thio relaxers and permanent waving is exactly the same.

_____ True

_____ False

112. The two most common types of hair relaxers are _____ and _____.

113. Extremely curly hair grows in long twisted spirals or coils, with the thinnest and weakest sections of the hair strands located at their twists.

_____ True

_____ False

114. _____ usually have a pH above 10 and a higher concentrate of ammonium thioglycolate than is used in permanent waving.

115. A relaxer can melt hair if it is used incorrectly.

_____ True

_____ False

116. The _____ used with thio relaxers is an oxidizing agent, usually hydrogen peroxide, just as in permanents.

117. A straightening process that involves thio relaxer and a flat iron is called

_____.

118. The _____ is the active ingredient in all hydroxide relaxers.

119. All hydroxide relaxers are very strong alkalis that can swell the hair up to twice its normal diameter.

_____ True

_____ False

120. Why are hydroxide relaxers not compatible with thio relaxers? _____

_____

121. Hydroxide relaxers remove one atom of sulfur from a disulfide bond, converting it into a lanthionine body by a process called _____.

122. The neutralization of hydroxide relaxers involves oxidation.

_____ True

_____ False

123. It is not possible to perm hair that has been treated with a _____.

124. _____ are ionic compounds formed by a metal—sodium (Na), potassium (K), or lithium (Li)—which is combined with oxygen (O) and hydrogen (H).

125. Sodium hydroxide relaxers are commonly called _____.

126. _____ and _____ relaxers are often advertised and sold as "no mix–no lye" relaxers.

127. _____ relaxers are usually advertised and sold as "no-lye" relaxers.

128. Guanidine hydroxide relaxers straighten the hair completely, with much less scalp irritation than other hydroxide relaxers.

_____ True

_____ False

129. _____ and _____ are sometimes used as low-pH hair relaxers.

130. _____ is an oily cream used to protect the skin and scalp during hair relaxing.

131. Why should base cream not touch the hair during the hair relaxing process?

_____.

132. _____ require the application of base cream to the entire scalp prior to the application of the relaxer.

133. _____ do not require application of a protective base. They contain a base cream that is designed to melt at body temperature.

134. List the different strengths of relaxers and what each is formulated for.

a) _____

b) _____

_____

c) _____

_____

135. One way to judge the timing of hair relaxing is to periodically perform a

_____.

136. _____ is used to deactivate the alkaline residues left in the hair by a hydroxide relaxer and lower the pH of the hair and scalp.

137. What does the application of an acid-balanced shampoo or normalizing lotion do? _____

_____

138. What hair straightening process requires special ventilation because it releases formaldehyde during the process? _____

_____

CURL RE-FORMING

139. What does curl re-forming accomplish? _____

_____

140. Before a client receives any permanent or hair-relaxing service, he or she should sign a(n) _____ that indicates he or she understand the possible _____ of the service.

CHAPTER 21 Haircoloring

Date: _____

Rating: _____

Text Pages: 626–684

POINT TO PONDER:

"The difference between a successful person and others is not a lack of strength, not a lack of knowledge, but rather a lack of will."—**Vince Lombardi**

WHY STUDY HAIRCOLORING?

1. How often do clients who color their hair usually visit the salon? _____

   _____

2. As a new cosmetologist, what are some of the important skills you should master before you begin applying color to your clients' hair?

   _____

   _____

   _____

   _____

3. One of the most creative, challenging, and popular salon services is _____.

4. Haircolor is both a _____ and an _____.

5. A skilled haircolorist needs to become an expert in what processes?

   a) _____

   b) _____

   c) _____

   d) _____

   e) _____

   f) _____

WHY PEOPLE COLOR THEIR HAIR

6. What are a few reasons clients color their hair?

a) _____

b) _____

c) _____

d) _____

_____

e) _____

7. Read the following sentences and decide if the missing term is *haircolor* or *hair color.*

John is mixing _____ for his client.

When Susan was young, her natural _____ was red.

Consuela had a bad experience with _____ she bought at the drugstore.

HAIR FACTS

8. What is the determining factor in choosing which haircolor to use that will affect the quality and ultimate success of the service? _____

9. Name and describe the three main parts of the hair.

a) _____

_____

b) _____

_____

c) _____

10. Which part of the hair contains the natural pigment? _____

11. The natural color of hair is determined by a substance called _____.

12. Hair _____ is determined by the diameter of the individual hair strand.

13. In fine hair the melanin granules are grouped more _____, so hair takes color _____ and can look darker.

14. Which hair type can take longer to process? _____

15. Hair _____ is the number of hairs per square inch (2.5 square cm), ranging from thin to thick.

16. _____ is the ability of the hair to absorb moisture.

17. Match each of the following degrees of porosity with its description.

_____ 1. Low porosity _____ 2. Average porosity _____ 3. High porosity	a) Cuticle is lifted; hair takes color quickly b) Cuticle is tight; hair is resistant c) Cuticle is slightly raised; hair is normal and processes in average amount of time

18. A strand of hair that feels smooth with a cuticle that is compact, dense, and hard has a _____ porosity.

19. Hair that is extremely _____ can process more quickly and result in a deeper hair color.

IDENTIFYING NATURAL HAIR COLOR AND TONE

20. What is the most important step in becoming a good colorist? _____

_____

21. The three main types of melanin in the cortex are:

a) _____

b) _____

c) _____

22. Natural hair color can be a combination of all types of melanin.

_____ True

_____ False

23. _____ is the pigment that lies under the natural hair color and must be taken into consideration when you select a haircolor. It is also known as

_____.

24. _____ is the unit of measurement used to identify the lightness or darkness of a color.

25. Haircolor levels are arranged on a scale of 1 to 10, with 1 being the _____ and 10 being the _____.

26. It is important for a cosmetologist to be able to identify degrees of lightness to darkness in each color level.

_____ True

_____ False

27. Gray hair is limited to the aging process.

_____ True

_____ False

28. Gray hair requires special attention in formulating haircolor.

_____ True

_____ False

29. What is salt-and-pepper hair? _____

_____

30. A person who has hair that is 70 to 90 percent gray usually has the most pigmented hair in which part of his or her head? _____

31. What are all colors developed from? _____

32. The _____ is a system for understanding color.

33. The law of color states that when combining colors, you will always get the same result from the same combination.

_____ True

_____ False

34. _____ are pure colors that cannot be achieved from a mixture.

35. The primary colors are _____.

36. _____ colors are created from the three primary colors.

_____ a) Some

_____ b) All

_____ c) Most

_____ d) A few

37. Colors with a predominance of blue are _____ colors, and colors with a predominance of red are _____ colors.

38. _____ is the strongest of the primary colors and is the only _____ primary color.

39. Which primary color can make other colors seem deeper or darker? _____

40. _____ is the medium primary color.

41. Red added to blue-based colors will cause them to appear:

_____ a) Darker

_____ b) Lighter

_____ c) Trendier

_____ d) Classic

42. Red added to yellow colors will cause them to become:

_____ a) Darker

_____ b) Lighter

_____ c) Trendier

_____ d) Classic

43. The weakest of the primary colors is _____.

44. When you add yellow to other colors, the resulting color will look:

_____ a) Deeper and darker

_____ b) Lighter and brighter

_____ c) More youthful

_____ d) More sophisticated

45. When all three colors are present in equal proportions, the resulting color depends on _____.

46. Which two colors cannot be made by mixing colors together?

a) _____

b) _____

47. A _____ color is a color obtained by mixing equal parts of two primary colors.

48. The secondary colors are _____.

49. Green is an equal combination of _____.

50. Orange is an equal combination of _____.

51. Violet is an equal combination of _____.

52. A _____ is an intermediate color achieved by mixing a secondary color and its neighboring primary color on the color wheel in _____ amounts.

53. Tertiary colors include:

a) _____

b) _____

c) _____

d) _____

e) _____

f) _____

54. _____ are a primary and secondary color positioned directly opposite each other on the color wheel.

55. Next to each of the following colors, list its complementary color.

Blue   _____

Red   _____

Yellow   _____

56. Complementary colors _____ each other.

57. Place a "P," "S," and "T" on the color wheel in their proper places to signify primary, secondary, and tertiary colors.

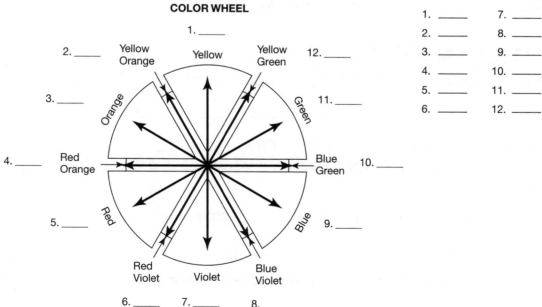

COLOR WHEEL

1. _____   7. _____
2. _____   8. _____
3. _____   9. _____
4. _____   10. _____
5. _____   11. _____
6. _____   12. _____

58. What color would you use to balance hair that is orange? _____

59. What color would you use to balance hair that is green? _____

60. What color would you use to balance hair that is yellow? _____

61. _____, or the hue of color, refers to the balance of the color and can be described as _____, _____, or _____.

62. _____ tones reflect light so they look lighter than the level they are. These tones are:

a) _____

b) _____

c) _____

d) _____

63. _____ tones are colors that absorb more light, so they look deeper than their actual level. These tones are:

a) _____

b) _____

c) _____

64. _____ tones are warm tones. They are described as _____ or _____.

65. A color can be as bright or as soft as desired; color _____ serve this purpose.

66. A _____ is the predominant tone of a color.

67. What base color is often used to cover gray hair? _____

TYPES OF HAIRCOLOR

68. What two categories do haircoloring products generally fall into? _____

_____

69. The oxidative category has two classifications: _____ _____; the nonoxidative category has two classifications: _____ _____.

70. What do all permanent haircolor products and lighteners contain? _____

_____

71. What are the three roles of ammonia or an ammonia substitute?

a) _____

_____

b) _____

c) _____

72. When the haircolor containing the alkalizing ingredient is combined with the developer, the peroxide becomes alkaline and decomposes or breaks up; lightening occurs when the alkaline peroxide breaks up the _____.

73. Temporary haircolor is a good choice for those who wish to _____ yellow hair or unwanted tones.

74. The pigments in _____ are large and do not penetrate the cuticle layer, allowing only a coating action that may be removed by _____.

75. Temporary haircolors are nonoxidation colors that make only a physical change, not a chemical change, in the hair shaft.

_____ True

_____ False

76. List the products that provide temporary hair color.

a) _____

_____

b) _____

c) _____

d) _____

e) _____

_____

77. _____ is formulated to last through several shampoos, depending on the hair's porosity.

78. How does semipermanent haircolor work? _____

_____

_____

_____

79. Semipermanent haircolor is required to be mixed with a peroxide.

_____ True

_____ False

80. How long does semipermanent color usually last? _____

_____

81. Demipermanent haircolor is also called _____. It is formulated to _____ but not lift, or lighten, color.

82. Demipermanent haircolor require both a high _____ and a high concentration of

_____.

83. What is a glaze? _____

84. No-lift deposit-only haircolors are ideal for:

a) _____

b) _____

c) _____

d) _____

85. No-lift deposit-only haircolor is available as a _____.

86. How long before a color service should a patch test be given?

_____ a) 12 to 24 minutes

_____ b) 24 to 48 minutes

_____ c) 12 to 24 hours

_____ d) 24 to 48 hours

87. _____ can lighten and deposit color at the same time in one process and are usually mixed with a higher-volume developer.

88. Permanent haircolor products generally contain uncolored dye precursors, also known as _____.

89. Dye precursors are small and can _____ into the hair shaft.

90. Molecules are trapped within the _____ of the hair and cannot be shampooed out.

91. What is a soap cap? _____

_____. When is it used? _____

_____

92. Permanent haircoloring products are regarded as the best products for covering _____ hair.

93. Permanent haircoloring simultaneously removes _____ from the hair through the action of lightening while adding _____ to both the gray and the pigmented hair.

94. Natural or _____ are natural colors obtained from the leaves or bark of plants. An example of this type of color is _____.

95. Do natural colors lighten the hair? _____

96. If a client who has used natural haircolor comes into the salon, can you apply additional chemical products over the top of natural haircolors? _____

97. _____, also called gradual colors, contain metal salts and change hair color gradually by progressive buildup and exposure to hair, creating a dull metallic appearance.

98. Historically, metallic haircolors been marketed to _____.

99. What are two drawbacks of metallic haircolor? _____

_____

100. A _____ is an oxidizing agent that, when mixed with an oxidative hair color, supplies the necessary oxygen gas to develop color molecules and create a change in hair color.

101. Developers are also called _____.

102. The pH of developer is:

_____ a) Between 1.0 and 2.3

_____ b) Between 2.5 and 4.5

_____ c) Between 6.5 and 7.5

_____ d) Between 8.5 and 9.5

103. Name the most commonly used developer on the market. _____

104. _____ measures the concentration and strength of hydrogen peroxide.

105. The lower the volume, the _____; the higher the volume, the

_____.

106. What happens if you apply haircolor with peroxide on hair that has been treated with metallic hair dye? _____

_____

107. Describe the common use of the following volumes of hydrogen peroxide.

a) 20 volume   _____

_____

b) 30 volume   _____

c) 40 volume   _____

_____

108. _____ lighten hair by dispersing, dissolving, and decolorizing the natural hair pigment.

109. What happens when hydrogen peroxide is mixed into the lightener formula? _____. The process is known as _____.

110. Hair lighteners are used to:

a) _____

b) _____

c) _____

d) _____

e) _____

111. How many stages of color may hair go through as it lightens?

_____ a) 3

_____ b) 5

_____ c) 8

_____ d) 10

112. Why would a colorist choose to decolorize a client's hair before tinting?

_____

_____

113. _____ are traditional semipermanent, demipermanent, and permanent haircolor products that are used primarily on prelighted hair to achieve pale and delicate colors after the _____ process.

114. All hair will go through all 10 degrees of decolorization.

_____ True

_____ False

115. How can you tell if you have damaged the hair during the decolorization process? _____

_____.

116. A person with dark hair will never be able to have pale blond hair.

_____ True

_____ False

CONSULTATION

117. A haircolor _____ is the most critical part of the color service.

118. During the consultation, your client will communicate _____ _____. It is important that you _____ so you can make an appropriate recommendation.

119. What is the single most reliable way to ensure a client's satisfaction? _____

_____

120. How much extra time should you book for a client consultation? _____ _____

121. Wall color should be _____ or _____ when performing the color consultation.

122. What is the purpose of the client information card? _____

_____

123. List some of the questions you might ask the client during the consultation.

a) _____

b) _____

c) _____

124. How many hair color options should you recommend to a client? _____ _____

125. Some medications may affect hair color.

_____ True

_____ False

126. A _____ is used by many salons when providing chemical services. Its purpose is to explain to clients that if their hair is in questionable condition, it may not withstand the requested chemical treatment.

127. Will a release statement clear the cosmetologist of responsibility for what may happen to a client's hair? _____

HAIRCOLOR FORMULATION

128. List the four basic questions you should ask when formulating a haircolor.

a) _____

b) _____

c) _____

d) _____

129. It is important to formulate with both _____ and _____ in mind.

130. List the two methods used for the application of permanent haircolor.

a) _____

b) _____

131. When using the brush and bowl technique, the bowl should be a _____ mixing bowl.

132. When working with haircolor, you will have to determine whether your clients have any allergies or sensitivities to the mixture. To do this you will administer a _____, also known as a _____.

133. How many hours prior to application of aniline haircolor should a patch test be given?

_____ a) 5 to 10

_____ b) 12 to 18

_____ c) 24 to 48

_____ d) 62 to 78

134. The color used for the patch test must be _____ _____.

135. A negative skin test result will show _____.

136. A positive skin test result will show _____.

HAIRCOLOR APPLICATIONS

137. A clearly defined system makes for the _____ and for the safest and most satisfactory results.

138. How can a colorist prevent colorist dermatitis? _____ _____

139. A _____ will tell you how the hair will react to the formula and how long the formula should be left on the hair.

140. When is the strand test performed? _____ _____

141. There is only one correct method for applying temporary haircolor.

_____ True

_____ False

142. Semipermanent colors do not contain the _____ necessary to lift. So they only _____.

143. When applying semipermanent color over existing color, remember that the color can _____ on the ends.

144. How is the application procedure for demipermanent haircolor determined?
_____

145. Why does gray hair present a challenge when formulating no-lift deposit-only haircolor? _____

_____

_____

146. How can you solve the problem discussed in Question 145? _____

_____

_____

147. Permanent haircolor applications are classified as either _____ -process or _____ -process.

148. _____ lightens and deposits color in a single application.

149. The first time the hair is colored is referred to as a _____.

150. A single-process tint that usually contains a nonammonia color and adds shine and tone to the hair is a _____.

151. As the hair grows, you will need to _____ to keep it looking attractive and to avoid a two-toned effect.

152. In a retouch, the tint should be applied to:

_____ a) The hair at the ends only

_____ b) The hair at the mid-shaft

_____ c) The new growth only

_____ d) The prelightened hair only

153. A visible line separating colored hair from new growth is called:

_____ a) Hyperpigmentation

_____ b) Hypopigmentation

_____ c) Line of demarcation

_____ d) Line of decolorization

154. What are some other names for hair lightening? _____

155. If a client asks for a dramatically lighter color, what has to be done? _____

_____

156. _____, also known as two-step coloring, is a technique requiring two separate procedures in which the hair is prelightened and then toned.

157. Why is a wider range of haircolor possible during a double-process high-lift coloring? _____

_____

USING LIGHTENERS

158. What are the three forms of lightener? _____

159. Oil and cream are _____, which can be used directly on the scalp.

160. New powder lighteners may also be used _____.

161. Why are on-the-scalp lighteners popular? _____

_____

162. List the features of cream lighteners.

a) _____

_____

b) _____

c) _____

_____

163. _____ contain a powdered oxidizer and/or the same persulfate salts that are used in powdered off-the-scalp hair lighteners.

164. _____ lighteners are strong enough for high-lift blonding, but gentle enough to be used on the scalp.

165. What does an activator do? _____

_____

166. How many activators can be used for on-the-scalp lightener applications?

_____

167. Too much heat used with a lightener will do what to hair? _____

_____

168. _____ are strong, fast-acting lighteners in powdered form.

169. Why should most powdered lighteners not be used for retouch services?

_____

170. Name the five factors that affect processing time for lighteners.

a) _____

_____

b) _____

c) _____

_____

d) _____

e) _____

171. To determine the processing time for your lightening service, the condition of the hair after lightening, and the end results, you should perform a _____ _____.

172. What is new growth? _____

_____

173. On a retouch, what should you lighten first?

_____ a) New growth

_____ b) Old growth

_____ c) It does not matter.

174. What will occur if lighteners are overlapped during a retouch? _____

_____

USING TONERS

175. Toners are used primarily on prelightened hair to achieve _____ colors.

176. What is most often used as a toner? _____

177. The _____ pigment is the color that remains in the hair after lightening.

178. As a general rule, the paler the color you are seeking, _____

_____.

179. Why should you not prelighten past the pale yellow stage? _____

_____

SPECIAL EFFECTS HAIRCOLORING

180. Special effects haircoloring refers to any technique that involves _____

_____.

181. Coloring some of the hair strands lighter than the natural color to add the illusion of depth is called _____.

182. Coloring strands of hair darker than the natural color is called _____

_____.

183. Name the three most frequently used techniques for achieving highlights.

a) _____

b) _____

c) _____

184. The _____ of highlighting involves pulling clean, dry strands of hair through a perforated cap with a thin plastic or metal hook.

185. The _____ of strands pulled through determines the degree of highlighting or lowlighting you can achieve.

186. The _____ of highlighting involves coloring selected strands of hair by slicing or weaving out sections, placing them on foil or plastic wrap, applying lightener or color, and sealing them in the foil or plastic wrap.

187. _____ involves taking a narrow, 1/8-inch (0.3 cm) section of hair by making a straight part at the scalp, positioning the hair over the foil, and applying lightener or color.

188. In _____, selected strands are picked up from a narrow section of hair with a zigzag motion of the comb, and lightener or color is applied only to these strands.

189. Name the four different patterns by which foil may be placed in the hair.

a) _____

b) _____

c) _____

d) _____

190. The _____ or the _____ technique involves the painting of a lightener directly onto clean, styled hair.

191. To avoid affecting untreated hair, you may choose:

a) _____

_____

b) _____

c) _____

_____

192. _____ are prepared by combining permanent haircolor, hydrogen peroxide, and shampoo.

193. When should you use a highlighting shampoo? _____

_____

194. Do you need to perform a patch test before using a highlighting shampoo?

_____

SPECIAL CHALLENGES IN HAIRCOLOR/CORRECTIVE SOLUTIONS

195. A skilled colorist will occasionally have a problem in haircolor that can't be predicted. This may be due to _____.

196. What can cause gray hair to have a yellow cast?

a) _____

b) _____

c) _____

d) _____

197. Which of the following should not be used to correct a yellow discoloration?

_____ a) Lightener

_____ b) Tint remover

_____ c) Violet-based colors

_____ d) Orange-based colors

198. Will hair color at a level 8 or lighter give complete gray coverage? Why or why not? _____

_____

199. Your client's hair is about 90 percent gray. Which color range would be most flattering to this client?

_____ a) Blond

_____ b) Red

_____ c) Black

200. What considerations should be taken into account when formulating haircolor for gray hair?

a) _____

b) _____

c) _____

201. List the tips for working with gray hair.

a) _____

b) _____

c) _____

d) _____

e) _____

f) _____

g) _____

h) _____

202. _____ raises the cuticle layer of gray or resistant hair to allow for better penetration of color.

203. List the rules for effective color correction.

a) _____

b) _____

c) _____

d) _____

e) _____

f) _____

g) _____

204. What are the characteristics of damaged hair?

a) _____

b) _____

c) _____

d) _____

e) _____

f) _____

205. When dealing with damaged hair, what should occur before proceeding with the chemical service? _____

206. When dealing with damaged hair:

a) _____

b) _____

_____

c) _____

d) _____

e) _____

207. _____ help equalize porosity.

208. The two main types of fillers are:

a) _____

b) _____

209. _____ fillers are used to recondition damaged, overly porous hair and equalize porosity.

210. _____ equalize porosity and deposit color in one application.

211. How do you select the right color filler to fix an unwanted haircolor? _____

_____

_____

212. A common problem with red haircolor is _____.

213. What color should natural highlights be in a brunette?

_____

214. What is the best way to achieve pale blond results?

_____

215. What might give hair a green cast?

_____

HAIRCOLORING SAFETY PRECAUTIONS

216. List the haircoloring safety precautions.

a) _____

_____

b) _____

c) _____

d) _____

e) _____

f) _____

g) _____

h) _____

i) _____

j) _____

k) _____

l) _____

m) _____

n) _____

22 Hair Removal

See Milady Standard Cosmetology Practical Workbook.

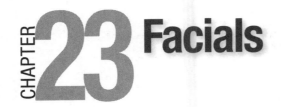

Date: _____

Rating: _____

Text Pages: 708–755

POINT TO PONDER:

"Change is inevitable. Growth is optional."—**Unknown**

WHY STUDY FACIALS?

1. Facial treatments can be very relaxing and offer many improvements to the
   _____ of the skin.

2. Proper skin care can make oily skin look _____; dry skin look
   and feel more _____; and aging skin look _____
   _____.

3. Why do you think it is important for you to learn the basics of skin analysis?

   _____

   _____

   _____

   _____

   _____

   _____

SKIN ANALYSIS AND CONSULTATION

4. _____ is a very important part of the facial treatment because it
   determines what type of the skin the client has, the condition of the skin, and
   what type of treatment the client's skin needs.

5. The opportunity to ask a client questions about his or her health and skin care
   history and to advise the client about appropriate home-care products and
   treatments occurs during the _____.

6. Why is it a good idea to perform cleaning and disinfection procedures in front of
   clients, whenever appropriate? _____

   _____

   _____

7. Before beginning the analysis, what must the client fill out? _____

_____

8. A(n) _____ is a condition the client has or a treatment the client is undergoing that might cause a negative side effect during a facial treatment.

9. Last week, your client Susan just stopped taking the drug isotretinoin for cystic acne. Today, she wants an exfoliation treatment. You should:

   _____ a) Provide the service as requested since she's now off the drug

   _____ b) Tell her she does not need an exfoliation

   _____ c) Explain that she needs to wait at least 6 months for this service

10. List the main contraindications to receiving a skin treatment you should look for on a client's completed health screening form

    a) _____

    _____

    b) _____

    c) _____

    d) _____

    e) _____

    f) _____

    g) _____

    h) _____

    i) _____

    j) _____

11. Which of the following services should not be performed on clients who are diabetic unless they have written approval from their physician? Check all that apply:

    _____ Waxing

    _____ Pedicure

    _____ Electrolysis

    _____ Makeup application

12. You may perform a facial on a client who has a fever blister, as long as you avoid the lip area.

    _____ True

    _____ False

13. If you know your client is prone to allergies, why do you need to check skin care products to see if they include food ingredients? _____

_____

_____

_____

14. What additional information can you obtain when the client completes the health screening form?

a) _____

b) _____

c) _____

d) _____

e) _____

_____

f) _____

15. Why should health screening forms be kept separately and secured?

_____

16. Why should you remove your rings or bracelets before performing a facial on a client? _____

_____

DETERMINING SKIN TYPE

17. It is possible to alter a client's skin type if you use the right product.

_____ True

_____ False

18. Skin that does not have obvious pores would be considered _____; another term for this type of skin is _____.

19. Clients with combination dry skin may have which of the following conditions?

_____ a) An orange peel texture to the skin

_____ b) A very smooth skin surface

_____ c) Clogged pores in the nose, chin, and center of the forehead

_____ d) Skin that appears tight and poreless

20. Why is acne considered a skin type? _____

_____

21. What are the two typical causes of hyperpigmentation of the skin?

_____

22. Acne is a disorder of the _____ that requires thorough and sometimes ongoing medical attention.

23. Generally, medical direction limits cosmetologists to the following measures in the treatment of acne:

a) _____

b) _____

c) _____

d) _____

24. Because acne skin contains infectious matter, you must wear protective gloves and use disposable materials.

_____ True

_____ False

SKIN CARE PRODUCTS

25. _____ are designed to clean the surface of the skin and to remove makeup.

26. List and describe the two types of cleansers.

a) _____

_____

b) _____

_____

27. Foaming cleansers contain surfactants, also known as _____, that cause the product to foam and rinse easily.

28. Toners, also known as _____ or _____, are designed to rebalance the pH of the skin after cleansing and to help remove excess cleansers from the skin.

29. Toners may contain ingredients that help to:

a) _____

b) _____

30. Fresheners and astringents are usually stronger products with higher _____ content and are used to treat _____.

31. How are toning products applied? _____

32. Some toners that contain alcohol may be sprayed on the face.

   _____ True

   _____ False

33. Cosmetologists are allowed to use products that remove dead surface cells from the _____.

34. Describe what exfoliants do. _____

35. What are exfoliants used for? _____

   _____

   _____

36. List the two basic types of exfoliants.

   a) _____

   b) _____

37. Mechanical exfoliants work by physically bumping off _____ buildup.

38. List some examples of mechanical exfoliants.

   a) _____

   b) _____

   c) _____

   d) _____

39. How do chemical exfoliants work? _____

40. Popular exfoliating chemicals are _____.

41. Describe how these acids work. _____

   _____

   _____

   _____

   _____

   _____

42. Salon alpha hydroxy acid (AHA) exfoliants are often referred to as _____.

43. How much AHA do they normally contain? _____

44. What are two precautions that must be taken before giving a client an AHA treatment?

a) _____

_____

b) _____

45. Some clients should not receive mechanical exfoliation or harsh mechanical peeling. List the five conditions that would contraindicate using these services on a client.

1) _____

2) _____

3) _____

_____

4) _____

_____

5) _____

46. _____ are another type of chemical exfoliant. They are known as _____ or protein-dissolving agents.

47. How does an enzyme peel work? _____

_____

48. Name the substance from which each enzyme has been made.

a) Papaya: _____

b) Pineapple: _____

c) Beef by-products: _____

49. What are the two basic types of keratolytic enzyme peels? _____

50. List the seven ways proper exfoliation may benefit a client's skin.

a) _____

b) _____

c) _____

d) _____

e) _____

f) _____

g) _____

51. Your client has particularly oily skin with many clogged pores. In this case it would be appropriate to use an exfoliant for a longer time period.

_____ True

_____ False

52. _____ are products that help increase the moisture content of the skin surface.

53. Moisturizers are mixtures of _____, also known as hydrators, which are oily or fatty ingredients that block moisture from leaving the skin.

54. What is an emollient? _____

_____

55. Moisturizers that are most often in lotion form and contain smaller amounts of emollient are for _____.

56. Moisturizers that are often in the form of a heavier cream and contain more emollients are for _____.

57. What is the most important habit to benefit the skin? _____

_____

58. A(n) _____ or higher is considered to be a thorough sunscreen strength.

59. Sun protection factor measures how _____ a person may be out in the sun without _____.

60. Night treatment products are usually more _____ products designed to be used at night to treat _____.

61. _____ and _____ are concentrated products that generally contain higher amounts of ingredients that have an effect on the skin appearance.

62. Lubricants to make the skin slippery during massage are called _____ _____.

63. What is a new product trend that is currently being seen in massage?

_____

64. _____ are products that are applied to the skin for a short time but have more immediate effects.

65. Match each type of mask with its intended use.

_____ 1. Clay-based masks	a) Used for dry skin; contain oils, emollients, and humectants; strong moisturizing effect
_____ 2. Cream masks	b) Melted at a little more than body temperature before application; harden to candle-like consistency
_____ 3. Gel masks	c) Contain special crystals of gypsum
_____ 4. Alginate masks	d) Used for oily and combination skin; generally oil-absorbing and have an exfoliating effect
_____ 5. Paraffin wax masks	e) Used for sensitive or dehydrated skin
_____ 6. Modelage masks	f) Often seaweed-based
_____ 7. Treatment cream	g) Applied underneath alginate masks

66. A thin, open-meshed fabric of loosely woven cotton is _____.

67. What is the purpose of gauze? _____

_____

68. _____ is sometimes used instead of gauze.

CLIENT CONSULTATION

69. All facial treatments should begin with a _____.

70. Why should the record card be kept at hand during the consultation?

_____

71. What should the record card contain?

a) _____

b) _____

c) _____

d) _____

_____

e) _____

_____

f) _____

_____

g) _____

h) _____

i) _____

_____

72. During the consultation, it is important to perform a thorough _____ _____ prior to cleansing.

73. Why should you always recommend beneficial services and products to clients?

_____

_____

_____

FACIAL MASSAGE

74. _____ is the manual or mechanical manipulation of the body by rubbing, gently pinching, kneading, tapping, and other movements.

75. What is the purpose of massage? _____

_____

76. Why do cosmetologists perform massage? _____

_____

77. To master massage techniques, you must have a basic knowledge of

_____.

78. Keep hands soft by using _____ and file and shape nails to avoid _____ your client.

79. The impact of a massage treatment depends on:

a) _____

b) _____

c) _____

80. The direction of movement is always from the _____ of the muscle toward its _____.

81. Which portion of the muscle is the more movable attachment, meaning it is attached to another muscle or a movable bone or joint? _____

82. Which portion of the muscle is the fixed attachment, meaning it is attached to an immovable section of the skeleton? _____

83. What could result if the muscle is massaged in the wrong direction? _____

_____

84. A cosmetologist should only massage which portions of a client's body?

a) _____

b) _____

c) _____

d) _____

e) _____

f) _____

g) _____

85. List the basic massage manipulations.

a) _____

b) _____

c) _____

d) _____

e) _____

f) _____

g) _____

h) _____

i) _____

j) _____

86. A client who has which of the following conditions should not have a facial massage?

_____ a) Diabetes

_____ b) Severe, uncontrolled hypertension

_____ c) Controlled high blood pressure

87. It is important to talk normally with your clients during a massage to help them feel more comfortable and relaxed.

_____ True

_____ False

88. Every muscle has a _____, which is a point on the skin over the muscle where pressure or stimulation will cause contraction of that muscle.

89. Identify the motor points on the illustration below:

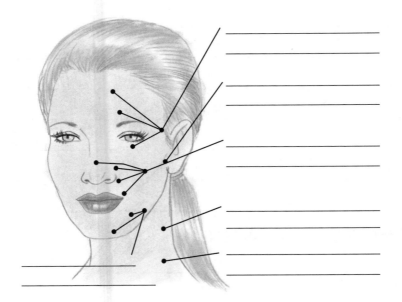

90. Identify the motor points on the illustration below:

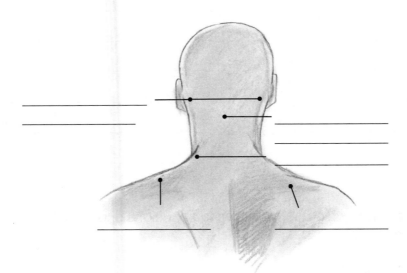

91. Relaxation is achieved through _____ or

_____.

92. The following benefits may be obtained by proper facial and scalp massage:

a) _____

b) _____

c) _____

d) _____

e) _____

f) _____

g) _____

93. Once you have started a facial massage do not _____ your hands from the client's face until you are done with the service.

94. What is an additional consideration required when massaging a male client's face?

_____

_____

_____

FACIAL EQUIPMENT

95. Never use facial equipment without first receiving _____ training and experience.

96. Facial machines will help to:

a) _____

b) _____

c) _____

97. A facial _____ heats and produces a stream of warm steam that can be focused on the client's face.

98. Steaming the skin helps to _____, making it more accepting of moisturizers and other treatment products. It also helps to _____ follicle accumulations such as comedones and clogged follicles.

99. When is steam usually administered? _____

_____

100. What may also be used for a steam treatment if a steamer is not available?

_____

_____

101. A rotating electric appliance with interchangeable brushes that can be attached to a rotating head is a(n) _____.

102. Brushing is a form of _____ and is usually administered after or during _____.

103. What does brushing do? _____

_____

104. Brushing should never be used on clients using _____ _____ or on clients who have _____ _____.

105. The skin suction and cold spray machine is used to _____ and to jet-spray lotions and toners onto the skin.

106. Skin suction should only be used on _____ and _____ skin.

107. Spray can be used on almost any skin type.

_____ True

_____ False

ELECTROTHERAPY AND LIGHT THERAPY

108. Galvanic and high-frequency treatment are types of _____, the use of electrical currents to treat the skin.

109. Electrotherapy should never be administered on:

a) _____

b) _____

c) _____

d) _____

e) _____

f) _____

g) _____

110. An _____ is an applicator for directing the electric current from the machine to the client's skin.

111. _____ machines have one electrode and _____ have two—a positive electrode called an _____, which has a red plug and cord, and a negative electrode called a _____, which has a black plug and cord.

112. The process of softening and emulsifying hardened sebum stuck in the follicles is known as _____.

113. _____ is the process that uses galvanic current to penetrate water-soluble products that contain ions into the skin.

114. It is critical to always apply the passive electrode on the _____ of the client's body to avoid having the current flow through the client's heart.

115. A type of galvanic treatment that is a computerized device that has many applications in skin care is _____.

116. _____ current is used to stimulate blood flow and help products penetrate.

117. Electrodes for high-frequency machines are made of _____.

118. How many electrodes do high-frequency machines require?

_____ a) 1

_____ b) 2

_____ c) 3

_____ d) 4

119. How can you prevent burns to a client during the use of galvanic current treatments? _____

_____

120. High frequency can be applied:

a) _____

b) _____

121. Traditionally, _____ have been used to heat the skin and increase blood flow.

122. What is the newest type of light therapy? _____

_____.

123. What does an LED treatment do? _____

_____

124. What is the cosmetic use of this newest form of light therapy? _____

_____

_____

_____

125. A client who has a(n) _____ disorder should not receive LED treatments.

126. A type of mechanical exfoliation that uses a closed vacuum to shoot crystals onto the skin, bumping off cell buildup that is then vacuumed by suction, is known as _____.

127. This treatment is used primarily to treat _____ and _____.

FACIAL TREATMENTS

128. Facial treatments fall into two categories:

a) _____

b) _____

129. Facial treatments help to:

a) _____

b) _____

c) _____

d) _____

e) _____

130. Home care is probably the most important factor in a successful skin care program. What is the key word in that statement? _____

131. Approximately how much time should you block out to explain proper home care to a client? _____

132. What does a skin care program consist of? _____

_____

AROMATHERAPY

133. Aromatherapy is the therapeutic use of _____, such as:

a) _____

b) _____

c) _____

134. Many essential oils are used for the aromatherapy benefits to enhance a person's _____.

135. It is beyond the scope of practice for a cosmetologist to perform _____ as part of aromatherapy.

136. Name three forms in which aromatherapy may be used in the salon.

a) _____

b) _____

c) _____

137. A caution when using essential oils is that too much can be _____.

24 Facial Makeup

Date: _____

Rating: _____

Text Pages: 756–790

POINT TO PONDER:

"It's easier to go down the mountain than up, but the view from the top is best."—**Unknown**

WHY STUDY FACIAL MAKEUP?

1. Makeup is a part of cosmetology that is very interesting and can produce _____ and _____ changes in the appearance.

2. Most clients prefer a _____, simply covering or focusing attention away from _____ and accenting good facial features.

3. Explain why you think it is important to know basic makeup techniques even if you plan to focus on providing hair and chemical services to clients.

   _____

   _____

   _____

   _____

COSMETICS FOR FACIAL MAKEUP

4. _____ is a tinted cosmetic, also known as _____, that is used to cover or even out the coloring of the skin.

5. Foundation can be used to _____

   _____.

6. Foundation is available in these three forms: _____.

7. A new trend in foundation is _____ makeup; this is a(n) _____ form of foundation.

8. Why would a color primer be applied to the skin? _____

   _____

9. A client who has a yellowish or sallow skin might benefit from which color primer?

_____ a) Green

_____ b) Amber

_____ c) Lavender

_____ d) Orange

10. Why would a skin primer be applied to the skin? _____

_____

11. Most liquid and cream foundations are mixtures of _____ spreading agents as a base containing a significant amount of talc and different coloring agents called _____.

12. Liquid foundations, also called _____ foundations, are mostly water but often contain an emollient such as mineral oil or a silicone such as cyclomethicone.

13. Water-based foundations are most often used for _____ and for oily to _____ skin types.

14. Which type of finish does a water-based foundation give to the skin? _____ What does this mean? _____

15. Foundations that are marketed as oil-free are usually intended for _____

_____.

16. Why do some oil-free foundations still make the skin look oily? _____

_____

17. _____, also known as oil-based, are considerably thicker products and are often sold in jars or tins.

18. Cream foundations always contain both oil and water.

_____ True

_____ False

19. Cream foundations provide _____ coverage and are usually intended for _____.

20. What will using cream foundations on oily or acneic skin cause? _____

_____

21. If a cosmetic product causes the formation of clogged pores or comedones, it is called _____, which means comedo-producing.

22. Some foundations also contain sunscreen.

_____ True

_____ False

23. Choosing the correct color of foundation is extremely important in _____

_____.

24. Foundation should be as close to a client's _____ as possible.

25. If the foundation is too light, how will it appear? _____

26. If the foundation is too dark, how will it appear? _____

27. How should foundation makeup be applied to the skin? _____

_____

28. What is a line of demarcation? _____

_____

29. _____ foundation contains a lot of pigment for coverage. The pigment sticks to the skin, providing a natural-looking coverage.

30. _____ are thicker and heavier types of foundation that contain more talc or pigment for heavier coverage.

31. What are concealers used for?

a) _____

b) _____

c) _____

32. Concealers are not available in a wide range of colors, and it may be difficult to match skin color.

_____ True

_____ False

33. What may happen if concealer color is not matched perfectly to skin tone?

_____

34. Some concealers may also contain ingredients that:

a) _____

b) _____

c) _____

35. A concealer may be worn without foundation.

_____ True

_____ False

36. Describe what you think are the most important considerations when choosing a foundation for a client.

_____

_____

_____

_____

_____

37. A cosmetic powder that is used to add a matte or nonshiny finish to the face is a(n) _____ .

38. List three uses for face powder.

a) _____

b) _____

c) _____

39. Face powder is available in two forms: _____ .

40. Pressed powder is blended with a _____ to keep it in a caked form in the tin. _____ does not contain as much binder and comes in a jar.

41. What are the three main ingredients in a face powder?

a) _____

b) _____

c) _____

42. Should powder puffs ever be used in the salon? Why? _____

_____

43. What is the purpose of cheek color? _____

_____

44. Is rouge different than blush? _____

_____

45. What forms does cheek color come in? _____

46. Name three places on the face where blush should not be applied.

a) _____

b) _____

c) _____

47. _____ is a paste-like cosmetic, usually in a metal or plastic tube, available in a large variety of colors and used to change or enhance the color of the lips.

48. Some lip color products contain conditioners to moisturize the lips or sunscreen to protect against sun exposure.

_____ True

_____ False

49. Lip color is available in a variety of forms including _____, _____, _____, _____, and _____.

50. Lip color must blend with a client's _____ and any other makeup that is used.

51. Fashion also helps dictate which of the following things about lipstick:

_____ a) Color

_____ b) Application styles

_____ c) Whether it looks shiny or matte

_____ d) All answers are correct.

52. When is it appropriate to apply lip color directly from its container? _____

_____

53. _____ is a colored pencil used to outline the lips and keep the lipstick from bleeding into small lines around the mouth.

54. Lip liner is usually applied before the lip color to _____.

55. How do you choose a lip liner color? _____

_____

56. _____ are cosmetics applied on the eyelids to accentuate or contour them.

57. Eye shadows are available in a variety of finishes, including:

a) _____

b) _____

c) _____

d) _____

e) _____

58. Eye shadows are available in:

a) _____

b) _____

c) _____

d) _____

59. Why should you avoid matching an eye shadow to a client's natural eye color?

_____

_____

60. A darker shade of eye color will have which effect?

_____ a) Make the natural color of the iris appear lighter

_____ b) Make the natural color of the iris appear darker

61. Match each of the following eye shadows with its description.

_____ 1. Base color	a) A shade lighter than the client's skin tone used to make an area appear larger
_____ 2. Contour color	b) A medium tone close to the client's skin tone
_____ 3. Highlight color	c) Deeper and darker than the client's skin tone

62. _____ is a cosmetic used to outline and emphasize the eyes.

63. Eyeliner is available in a variety of colors, in pencil, _____, pressed, or felt-tip pen form.

64. What does eyeliner do? _____

65. Eyeliner pencils consist of a wax _____ or hardened oil-base _____ with a variety of additives to create color.

66. Most clients prefer to use an eyeliner color that is the same color as their _____.

67. Where should you not apply eyeliner?

_____ a) Close to the lash line on the top eyelid

_____ b) Below the lash line on the bottom eyelid

_____ c) On the inner rim of the eyes

68. _____ are used to add color to the eyebrows, usually after tweezing or waxing.

69. Besides adding color, what are two reasons to use an eyebrow pencil?

a) _____

b) _____

70. _____ is a cosmetic preparation used to darken, define, and thicken the eyelashes.

71. Mascara is available in _____ forms.

72. What are the most popular shades for mascara? _____

73. Name six ingredients that are contained in mascara.

a) _____

b) _____

c) _____

d) _____

e) _____

f) _____

74. _____ remove eye makeup products that are water-resistant.

75. _____ is a heavy makeup used for theatrical purposes.

76. A shaped, solid mass applied to the face with a moistened cosmetic sponge is

_____ .

77. Match each of the following makeup tools with its description.

_____ 1. Powder brush	a) Used to remove excess facial hair
_____ 2. Concealer brush	b) Used to give lift and upward curl to the upper lashes
_____ 3. Eyeliner brush	c) Brush with firm, thin bristles
_____ 4. Angle brush	d) Large, soft brush used to apply powder and for blending edges of color.
_____ 5. Tweezers	e) Narrow, firm brush with a flat edge
_____ 6. Eyelash curler	f) Brush with fine, tapered, firm bristles

MAKEUP COLOR THEORY

78. _____ are fundamental colors that cannot be obtained from a mixture.

79. The primary colors are _____, _____, and _____.

80. _____ are obtained by mixing equal parts of two primary colors.

81. _____ are obtained by mixing equal amounts of a secondary color and its neighboring primary color on the color wheel.

82. Orange is made by mixing _____ and _____.

83. Green is made by mixing _____ and _____.

84. Violet is made by mixing _____ and _____.

85. A primary and secondary color directly opposite each other on the color wheel are called _____.

86. When mixed, complementary colors cancel each other out to create a _____ _____ color.

87. When placed next to each other, complementary colors will _____
_____.

88. _____ are the range of colors from yellow and gold through the oranges, red-oranges, most reds, and even some yellow-greens.

89. _____ suggest coolness and are dominated by blues, greens, violets, and blue-reds.

90. What is a neutral skin tone? _____
_____

91. Your client has dark skin and wants her makeup to look subtle. You would therefore use:

_____ a) Light colors

_____ b) Medium colors

_____ c) Dark colors

92. Neutral makeup with an orange-brown tone would be considered:

_____ a) Warm

_____ b) Cool

93. A complementary color for brown eyes is _____
_____.

94. A complementary color for blue eyes is _____

_____ .

95. Why is it not recommended to mix both warm and cool colors on the face?

_____

_____

96. The choice of color for eye makeup also depends on a person's _____ .

BASIC PROFESSIONAL MAKEUP APPLICATION

97. The first step in the makeup process is the _____ .

98. You should _____ and try not to impose your own opinions too much.

99. The consultation area must be _____ .

100. Describe the type of lighting that is required for a makeup consultation area.

_____

_____

_____

101. Which form of artificial light is more flattering?

_____ a) Fluorescent light

_____ b) Incandescent light

102. What information should you record on the consultation card?

a) _____

b) _____

c) _____

d) _____

e) _____

f) _____

g) _____

SPECIAL-OCCASION MAKEUP

103. What type of makeup is most appropriate for a client who is going to be photographed frequently, such as at a wedding? _____

104. Your client has fantastic eyes, cheekbones, and lips. How should you approach applying her makeup for a special occasion?

_____ a) Play up her lips, eyes, and cheekbones so she looks great

_____ b) Intensify two of these features to help them stand out

_____ c) Focus on minimizing her flaws; her positive features don't need your help

_____ d) None of these answers are correct.

105. Which colors tend to work best on older clients who have many wrinkles?

_____ a) Softer colors

_____ b) Frosted colors

_____ c) Shimmering colors

CORRECTIVE MAKEUP

106. Creative makeup techniques are used to _____

_____.

107. Facial features can be _____ with proper highlighting, _____ with correct shadowing or shading, and _____ with the proper hairstyle.

108. The basic rule of makeup application is to _____

_____.

109. A basic rule for makeup application is the following: Use a highlight to _____ a feature; use a shadow to _____ a feature.

110. Before you apply corrective makeup on a client, you must know how to _____ face shapes.

111. Match each of the following face shapes with its description.

_____ 1. Oval	a. Narrow forehead with wide cheekbones
_____ 2. Round	b. Usually three-fourths as long as it is wide
_____ 3. Square	c. Also called heart-shaped
_____ 4. Triangular	d. Rounded chin and hairline
_____ 5. Inverted triangle	e. Jaw is wider than the forehead
_____ 6. Diamond	f. Long, narrow face
_____ 7. Oblong	g. Wide forehead and square jawline

112. What is the best way to conceal a protruding nose? _____

_____

_____

113. What is the best way to conceal a broad nose? _____

_____

_____

114. What is the best way to conceal a double chin? _____

_____

115. What is the best way to enhance close-set eyes? _____

_____

116. How can you use makeup to make small eyes seem larger? _____

_____

117. What colors work best with deep-set eyes? _____

118. How should color be applied to close-set eyes? _____

_____

119. A person who has over-tweezed eyebrows may look _____.

120. How can eyebrow shape help make wide-set eyes seem closer together?

_____

121. A high arch at the ends of the eyebrows will help a _____ face appear more oval.

122. What is Latisse? _____

_____

123. How can you minimize wrinkles that are due to dry skin? _____

_____

_____

ARTIFICIAL EYELASHES

124. Why has the use of artificial eyelashes grown enormously?

a) _____

b) _____

125. What is the objective of artificial eyelashes? _____

_____

126. _____, also called strip lashes, are eyelash hairs on a strip that are applied with adhesive to the natural lash line.

127. _____ are separate artificial eyelashes that are applied to the eyelids one at a time.

128. _____ is the product used to make artificial eyelashes adhere to the natural lash line.

129. Why should a client avoid getting artificial lashes wet? _____

_____

130. Some clients may be allergic to eyelash adhesive.

_____ True

_____ False

CHAPTER 25 Manicuring

See Milady Standard Cosmetology Practical Workbook.

CHAPTER 26 Pedicuring

See Milady Standard Cosmetology Practical Workbook.

CHAPTER 27 Nail Tips and Wraps

See Milady Standard Cosmetology Practical Workbook.

CHAPTER 28 Monomer Liquid and Polymer Powder Nail Enhancements

See Milady Standard Cosmetology Practical Workbook.

CHAPTER 29 UV Gels

See Milady Standard Cosmetology Practical Workbook.

30 Seeking Employment

Date: _____

Rating: _____

Text Pages: 956–983

POINT TO PONDER:

"The ability to concentrate and to use your time well is everything."
—Lee Iacocca

WHY STUDY HOW TO PREPARE FOR AND SEEK EMPLOYMENT?

1. Making the wrong job choice may cause _____ in starting your career.

2. Passing the State Board exam and obtaining your license is optional in most states.

   _____ True

   _____ False

3. Describe two skills you will need to master to find a secure job in a salon.

   _____

   _____

   _____

PREPARING FOR LICENSURE

4. List the five factors that will affect how well you perform during the licensing examination or on tests in general.

   a) _____

   b) _____

   c) _____

   d) _____

   _____

   e) _____

5. Being _____ means understanding the _____ for successfully taking tests.

6. A test-wise student prepares for taking a test by practicing _____ and _____.

7. List the daily habits and time management skills of effective studying.

a) _____

b) _____

c) _____

d) _____

e) _____

f) _____

g) _____

h) _____
   _____

8. What holistic steps can you take to prepare for test taking?

a) _____
   _____

b) _____

c) _____

d) _____

e) _____

f) _____
   _____

9. What strategies can you adapt on test day?

a) _____

b) _____

c) _____
   _____

d) _____
   _____

e) _____

_____

f) _____

g) _____

_____

h) _____

i) _____

_____

j) _____

_____

_____

k) _____

l) _____

_____

m) _____

_____

n) _____

_____

o) _____

p) _____

_____

10. _____ is the process of reaching logical conclusions by employing logical reasoning.

11. When taking a test, you should begin by eliminating options you know are incorrect.

_____ True

_____ False

12. Study the _____, or the _____, because it will often provide a clue to the correct answer.

13. Give three examples of qualifying conditions or statements you might find in a test question.

a) _____

b) _____

c) _____

14. In reading-type tests that contain long paragraphs followed by several questions, read the _____ first. This will help identify the _____ elements in the paragraph.

15. The most important strategy of test taking is to _____.

16. In true/false questions look for qualifying words such as _____ _____; absolutes are generally _____.

17. In a true/false statement, only part of the statement needs to be true.

_____ True

_____ False

18. Short statements are more likely to be true than longer ones.

_____ True

_____ False

19. When taking a multiple choice test, read the entire question carefully, including all the _____.

20. When answering multiple choice questions, it is wise to eliminate completely incorrect answers first.

_____ True

_____ False

21. Keep in mind that when two multiple choice answers seem similar, one of them is likely to be the _____ answer.

22. In multiple choice questions, the answer choice "All of the above" is often the correct answer.

_____ True

_____ False

23. When answering matching questions, it is best to read all items in each list before beginning.

_____ True

_____ False

24. What strategy can you use when answering matching questions to help yourself?

_____

25. When answering essay questions, make sure that what you write is

_____, _____, _____, _____,

and _____ .

26. To be successful at test taking, you must follow the rules of _____ and be _____ of the exam content for both the practical and written examination.

27. To better prepare for the practical portion of the exam, you should:

a) _____

b) _____

_____

c) _____

_____

d) _____

_____

e) _____

_____

f) _____

_____

g) _____

_____

h) _____

_____

i) _____

_____

j) _____

_____

PREPARING FOR EMPLOYMENT

28. Answer the following questions in your own words.

a) What do you really want out of a career in cosmetology?

_____

_____

b) What particular areas within the beauty industry interest you most?

_____

_____

_____

c) What are your strongest practical skills, and in what ways do you wish to use them? _____

_____

_____

d) What personal qualities will help you have a successful career?

_____

_____

_____

29. Willingness to work hard is a key ingredient to your _____.

30. List the key personal characteristics that will help you get and keep the position you want.

a) _____

b) _____

c) _____

d) _____

e) _____

31. "The best kind of motivation is internal." Explain why you agree or disagree with this statement.

_____

_____

_____

_____

_____

_____

32. People who care about the quality and consistency of their job performance are said to have a _____ .

33. Match the following type of salon with the phrase that best describes it.

_____ 1. Small independent salon

a) Chains of five or more salons that are owned by one individual

_____ 2. Independent salon chain

b) Chain salon organization; one with a national name, owned by individuals who pay a fee to use the name

_____ 3. Large national salon chain

c) Salon owned by an individual or two or more partners

_____ 4. Franchise salon

d) Company operates salons throughout the country

34. Match the following type of salon with the phrase that best describes it.

_____ 1. Value-priced salons

a) Salons that offer luxurious, higher-priced services and treatments

_____ 2. Full-service salons

b) Salons that depend on high volume of traffic and charge low prices

_____ 3. Image salons

c) Salons that offer a complete menu of hair, nail, and skin care services

35. A recent cosmetology graduate is most likely to easily find a job in a(n) _____ .

36. What is possibly the least expensive way of owning one's own business?

_____

37. What guidelines should you follow when preparing your professional resume?

a) _____

b) _____

c) _____

_____

d) _____

e) _____

_____

f) _____

g) _____

38. The average potential employer will spend _____ scanning your resume before deciding whether or not to grant you an interview.

39. When writing a resume, you should focus on your _____.

40. List the do's and don'ts of resumes.

Do's:

a) _____

b) _____

c) _____

d) _____

e) _____

f) _____

g) _____

h) _____

i) _____

j) _____

k) _____

l) _____

Don'ts:

a) _____

b) _____

c) _____

41. When you are marketing yourself for a job, think of yourself as a(n) _____ , not just a resume.

42. A(n) _____ is a collection of photos and documents that reflects your skills, accomplishments, and abilities in your chosen career.

43. A powerful portfolio includes:

a) _____

b) _____

c) _____

d) _____

e) _____

_____

f) _____

g) _____

h) _____

_____

i) _____

j) _____

44. Once you have created your employment portfolio, it is a good idea to:

_____ a) Not look at it again for a while.

_____ b) Show it to a neutral party for feedback.

_____ c) Mail it to all of the salons in your area.

45. Why is it a good idea to mention that you work well as a member of a team when you prepare your statement about why you chose a career in cosmetology?

_____

_____

_____

_____

46. List the points to consider when narrowing your job search for the best possible results.

a) _____

b) _____

c) _____

d) _____

_____

e) _____

f) _____

g) _____

_____

47. A great way to find out about jobs is to actually _____ .

48. _____ allows you to establish contacts that may eventually lead to a job and helps you gain valuable information about the workings of various establishments.

49. List the guidelines to follow when networking with local salons.

a) _____

b) _____

c) _____

_____

d) _____

_____

e) _____

_____

f) _____

_____

50. When is it appropriate to text a salon owner or manager of a salon where you would like to work someday?

_____ a) Always; this is more effective than calling.

_____ b) Never; this is considered rude.

_____ c) It depends; if they say it is OK, then do it.

51. If a salon rejects your request to visit, it means you have done something wrong.

_____ True

_____ False

52. When you visit a salon, take your _____ to ensure that you observe all the key areas that might affect your decision making.

53. After visiting a salon, remember to _____

_____.

54. Why is it important to build relationships with salons you visit, even if you decide you do not want to work there?

_____

_____

THE JOB INTERVIEW

55. When you decide to make contact with an appropriate salon to ask for an interview, you should send only your resume.

_____ True

_____ False

56. You see a job you like on a salon's Web site. How should you apply for it?

_____

_____

_____

57. How soon after applying for a position should you follow up with a salon?

_____ a) The next day

_____ b) A week later

_____ c) A month later

58. When preparing for an interview, make sure you have all the following items in place:

a) _____

b) _____

c) _____

d) _____

e) _____

59. How many interview outfits should you have? _____

60. Your interview outfit should be _____ for the position for which you are applying.

61. Before going on an interview, make sure both your hairstyle and makeup are _____.

62. What supporting materials should you also have in place?

a) _____

b) _____

c) _____

63. The following questions are typical of ones you may be asked during an interview. To prepare yourself for job interviews, answer the questions now.

_____

_____

a) Why do you want to work here? _____

_____

b) What did you like best about your training? _____

_____

c) Are you punctual and regular in attendance? _____

_____

d) Will your school director or instructor confirm this? _____

_____

e) What skills do you feel are your strongest? _____

_____

f) What areas do you consider yourself to be less strong in? _____

_____

g) Are you a team player? Please explain. _____

_____

_____

h) Do you consider yourself flexible? Please explain. _____

_____

_____

i) What are your career goals? _____

_____

_____

j) What days and hours are you available for work? _____

_____

_____

k) Are there any obstacles that would prevent you from keeping your commitment to full-time employment? _____

_____

_____

l) What assets do you believe that you would bring to this salon and this position? _____

_____

_____

m) What computer skills do you have? _____

_____

_____

n) How would you handle a problem client? _____

_____

_____

o) How do you feel about retailing? _____

_____

_____

p) Would you be willing to attend our company training program? _____

_____

_____

q) Describe ways that you provide excellent customer service. _____

_____

_____

r) Please share an example of consultation questions that you might ask a
client. _____

_____

_____

s) Are you prepared to train for a year before you get your own clients? _____

_____

_____

64. Some salons require job interviewees to _____ as part of the
interview.

65. What should you bring with you to the interview if you will have to perform a
service? _____

66. What behaviors should you practice in connection with the interview?

a) _____

b) _____

_____

c) _____

d) _____

e) _____

f) _____

g) _____

h) _____

i) _____

j) _____

k) _____

l) _____

m) _____

n) _____

67. List some questions that you might consider asking during a job interview.

a) _____

b) _____

c) _____

d) _____

e) _____

f) _____

g) _____

h) _____

i) _____

j) _____

_____

k) _____

l) _____

m) _____

n) _____

68. Next to each question, indicate whether it is legal or illegal to ask in an interview:

a) How old are you?   _____

b) Would you describe your medical   _____
   history?

c) Are you over the age of 18?   _____

d) Are you able to perform this job?   _____

e) Are you a U.S. citizen?   _____

f) Are you authorized to work in the   _____
   United States?

g) In which languages are you fluent?   _____

69. A non compete contract prevents you from seeking other employment for a given amount of _____.

70. A salon manager offers you a job on the spot, then hands you a non compete contract. What is the best way for you to handle this?

_____ a) Accept the job happily and sign the contract immediately

_____ b) Explain that you refuse to sign a non compete contract

_____ c) Say "thank you" and ask for a few days to think things over

71. Once employed, take the necessary steps to learn all you can about your new position by:

a) _____

b) _____

c) _____

31 On the Job

Date: _____

Rating: _____

Text Pages: 984–1005

POINT TO PONDER:

"You cannot always have happiness, but you can always give happiness."—**Unknown**

WHY STUDY WHAT IT IS LIKE ON THE JOB?

1. Working in a salon means you are a member of a(n) _____.

2. What does the term *financial management* mean to you? Why do you think it is important to understand this as a salon professional?

_____

_____

_____

_____

_____

_____

_____

_____

MOVING FROM SCHOOL TO WORK

3. Once you become the employee of a salon, you are expected to put the needs of the _____ ahead of your own.

4. Putting the salon and the clients' needs first means:

a) _____

b) _____

OUT IN THE REAL WORLD

5. In a job, you will never have to do any work or perform services that aren't what you want to do.

    _____ True

    _____ False

6. To be successful, you must determine the position that is _____.

7. The number one thing to remember when you are in a service business is that your work revolves around _____.

8. List the five key points to remember in serving others.

    a) _____

    b) _____

    c) _____

    d) _____

    e) _____

9. Working in a salon requires that you practice and perfect your _____ and become a good _____.

10. List the habits of successful team players.

    a) _____

    b) _____

    c) _____

    d) _____

    e) _____

    f) _____

    g) _____

    h) _____

11. When you take a job, you will be expected to:

    a) _____

    b) _____

    c) _____

12. A document that outlines all the duties and responsibilities of a particular position in a salon or spa is a _____.

13. If your salon does not have a job description, you may want to _____

_____.

14. If you are unclear about something, you should _____.

15. A job description should cover:

a) _____

b) _____

c) _____

16. The three standard methods of compensation in a salon are _____,

_____, and _____.

17. An excellent source of affordable continuing education courses may be found on the _____.

18. An hourly rate is generally offered to a new practitioner and is usually based on

_____.

19. A _____ may be offered to you instead of an hourly rate; it should be at least equal to the _____ for the number of hours you work.

20. A _____, a percentage of the revenue that the salon takes in from its sales, is usually offered to practitioners once they have built up a loyal clientele.

21. Commissions are paid on your total _____.

22. Commissions range anywhere from 25 percent to 60 percent and are usually based on:

a) _____

b) _____

c) _____

23. A salary-plus-commission structure basically means that you receive both a _____ and a _____.

24. Another name for a salary-plus-commission is _____.

25. This kind of structure is commonly used to _____ practitioners to perform more services.

26. It is customary for salon professionals to receive _____ from satisfied clients.

27. The standard amount of a tip is usually _____ of the total service ticket.

28. A tip for a service that cost $60 would be:

_____ a) $6.00

_____ b) $7.50

_____ c) $9.00

29. Tips must be reported as income.

_____ True

_____ False

30. An _____ is the best way to keep tabs on your progress and to get feedback from your salon manager and key coworkers.

31. Commonly, evaluations are scheduled _____ days after hiring and then once a year after that.

32. Ask a _____ to sit in on one of your client consultations and make note of areas where you can improve.

33. One of the best ways to improve your performance is to model your behavior after someone who is having the kind of success you wish to have and to use that person as a _____.

34. When seeking out a role model, observe a stylist who is really good and determine:

a) _____

b) _____

c) _____

d) _____

e) _____

_____

f) _____

g) _____

35. What should you do if your mentor sees things differently than you do? _____

_____

MANAGING YOUR MONEY

36. A career in the beauty industry is very _____; it is also a career that requires _____ and planning.

37. The best way to meet all of your financial responsibilities is to know _____ _____, so you can make informed decisions about where your money goes.

38. The term that means not paying back your loans is called _____.

39. One step to ensure that you always have enough money is _____ _____.

40. What are three ways you may be able to use technology to help your salon and show you are technologically savvy?

a) _____

b) _____

c) _____

41. A good way to manage and keep track of your money is to create a personal _____.

42. How can you generate greater income for yourself?

a) _____

b) _____

c) _____

d) _____

e) _____

43. To get help with personal finances, you should seek the advice of a personal _____, who will be able to give you advice on reducing your credit card debt, investing your money, and retirement options.

DISCOVER THE SELLING YOU

44. The practice of recommending and selling additional services to your clients is called _____ or _____.

45. When you recommend additional salon services, you will always be the one who performs them on your client.

_____ True

_____ False

46. _____ is the act of recommending and selling products to your clients for at-home hair, skin, and nail care.

47. To be successful in sales, you need:

a) _____

b) _____

c) _____

48. What is the first step in selling? _____

49. List the principles of selling.

a) _____

_____

b) _____

_____

c) _____

d) _____

_____

e) _____

f) _____

_____

g) _____

_____

h) _____

50. A _____ involves informing clients about a product, without stressing they purchase it. A _____ approach focuses emphatically on why clients should buy the product.

51. What are the various reasons clients are motivated to buy salon products?

a) _____

b) _____

c) _____

52. Your first consideration is to always keep in mind the _____.

53. To sell a product, you will need to understand a client's _____ and how they may be _____.

54. How can you get the conversation started on retailing products?

a) _____

_____

b) _____

c) _____

d) _____

_____

e) _____

f) _____

g) _____

_____

h) _____

KEEPING CURRENT CLIENTS AND EXPANDING YOUR CLIENT BASE

55. Once you have mastered the basics of good service, take a look at some _____ that will keep your clients coming back to you.

56. List suggested marketing techniques that will keep your clients coming back to you.

a) _____

b) _____

c) _____

d) _____

57. What things can you do to build your client base?

a) _____

b) _____

c) _____

d) _____

e) _____

58. List five key points you should keep in mind when selling products or services to clients.

a) _____

b) _____

c) _____

d) _____

e) _____

59. The best time to think about getting your client back into the salon is while she or he is still in your salon.

_____ True

_____ False

60. The best way to encourage your clients to book another appointment before they leave is to _____

_____ .

ON YOUR WAY

61. Both new stylists and those who have been working in the business for a while should always remain willing to _____ .

62. Remember, your _____ job is most likely to be your most _____ one.

32 The Salon Business

Date: _____

Rating: _____

Text Pages: 1006–1030

POINT TO PONDER:

"He who does not get fun and enjoyment out of every day . . . needs to reorganize his life."—**George Matthew Adams**

WHY STUDY THE SALON BUSINESS?

1. To be successful in the beauty industry, you should be prepared to be two things: a(n) _____ and a(n) _____.

2. Most salon owners have worked as stylists.

    _____ True

    _____ False

3. You have no future plans to own your own business. Why is it still important for you to understand the rules of business that affect salons?

    _____

    _____

    _____

    _____

    _____

GOING INTO BUSINESS FOR YOURSELF

4. The two main options for being your own boss are:

    a) _____

    b) _____

5. Salon owners do not usually work on clients of their own.

    _____ True

    _____ False

6. Another term for booth rental is _____.

7. In a booth rental arrangement, a practitioner generally:

a) _____

b) _____

_____

c) _____

d) _____

8. Booth rental is a desirable situation for _____

_____.

9. What are the obligations of renting a booth?

a) _____

b) _____

c) _____

d) _____

e) _____

f) _____

g) _____

_____

h) _____

i) _____

j) _____

_____

k) _____

l) _____

_____

m)_____

10. Which state does not currently allow booth rental? _____

11. As a booth renter, you will not enjoy the same benefits as an employee of a salon would, such as _____.

12. What is a vision statement? _____

_____

13. How is a mission statement different from a vision statement?

_____

_____

_____

_____

_____

14. A set of benchmarks that help business owners achieve their mission and vision is called _____.

15. What portion of the business timeline is devoted to tending to business, its clientele, and its employees?

_____ a) Year One

_____ b) Years Two to Five

_____ c) Years Five to Ten

_____ d) Years Eleven to Twenty

16. Why is the name you choose for your salon important?

1) _____

2) _____

_____

3) _____

17. List the basic factors to carefully consider when opening a salon.

a) _____

b) _____

c) _____

d) _____

e) _____

f) _____

g) _____

h) _____

18. What are the elements of a good business location? _____

_____

19. A(n) _____ is a written description of your business as you see it today and as you foresee it in the next 5 years.

20. A business plan is legally binding once you have signed it.

_____ True

_____ False

21. What should be included in your business plan?

a) _____

b) _____

c) _____

d) _____

e) _____

22. What is meant by area demographics? _____

_____

23. You may call on the services of a(n) _____ to help you gather accurate financial information.

24. What kind of laws must be complied with when you open a salon?

_____

25. You must also comply with federal _____ _____ guidelines to ensure you are operating your salon in compliance with safety regulations.

26. What kinds of insurance must you purchase when you open your own business?

_____

27. What are salon policies? _____

_____

_____

28. What are the three types of ownership?

a) _____

b) _____

c) _____

29. Describe a business that is owned by a sole proprietor. _____

_____

_____

_____

30. Describe a partnership. _____

_____

_____

_____

31. Describe a business owned by a corporation. _____

_____

_____

32. What is capital? _____

33. What is a franchise? _____

_____

_____

_____

34. It is important that all franchise locations:

_____ a) Are run the same way

_____ b) Carry different products

_____ c) Look differently

35. Choosing to run a franchise will guarantee you are successful.

_____ True

_____ False

36. List the eight parts of a business plan.

a) _____

b) _____

c) _____

d) _____

e) _____

f) _____

g) _____

h) _____

37. If you choose to purchase an existing salon, your agreement to purchase should
include:

a) _____

_____

b) _____

c) _____

_____

d) _____

_____

_____

e) _____

f) _____

g) _____

_____

h) _____

_____

i) _____

_____

38. A lease should specify the following:

a) _____

_____

b) _____

_____

c) _____

_____

39. What can you do to protect your salon against fire, theft, and lawsuits?

a) _____

_____

b) _____

_____

c) _____

_____

d) _____

_____

_____

e) _____

_____

40. To run a people oriented business you need:

a) _____

b) _____

41. Smooth business management depends on the following factors:

a) _____

b) _____

c) _____

d) _____

e) _____

f) _____

g) _____

h) _____

42. As a business operator, you must always know where your money

_____.

43. Proper _____ are necessary to meet the needs of local, state, and federal laws regarding taxes and employees.

44. _____ is classified as receipts from service and retail sales.

45. _____ include rent, utilities, insurance, salaries, advertising, equipment, and repairs.

46. _____ help establish the net worth of a business at the end of the year.

47. Supplies that are used in the daily business operation are _____, and those to be sold to clients are _____.

48. A good way to keep track of service records or client cards is by using a(n) _____.

OPERATING A SUCCESSFUL SALON

49. How can you ensure that you will stay in business and have a prosperous salon?

_____

50. When planning a salon's layout, maximum _____ should be the primary concern.

51. If you plan to include a spa as part of your business, the spa area should be _____ from the service area.

52. The retail area in an upscale salon should be spacious, _____, and well lit.

53. Ideally, you should consult with a(n) _____ to help you plan the layout of your salon.

54. About how long does it normally take a new salon to begin operating at full capacity? _____

55. The term *personnel* refers to a salon's _____ or _____.

56. What determines the number of salon employees? _____

57. When interviewing potential employees, consider the following:

a) _____

b) _____

c) _____

d) _____

e) _____

58. What are some ways you can share your success with your staff?

a) _____

b) _____

c) _____

d) _____

e) _____

f) _____

_____

g) _____

59. It is not possible to learn how to manage other people; this is a skill that must come naturally to a manager.

_____ True

_____ False

60. Name two important civil rights laws all employers must be familiar with.

1) _____

2) _____

61. The best salons employ professional _____ to handle the job of scheduling appointments and greeting clients.

62. The reception area should be _____.

63. The receptionist should be _____
_____.

64. The receptionist handles important functions such as:

a) _____

b) _____

c) _____

d) _____

e) _____

65. What additional tasks will a receptionist perform in the salon during slow periods? _____
_____

66. Appointments must be scheduled to make the most efficient use of everyone's

_____.

67. A receptionist must have the following qualities:

a) _____

a) _____

a) _____

68. The appointment book may be an actual book that sits atop the reception desk, or it may be a _____ appointment book.

69. A major part of the salon business is handled over the _____.

70. When using the telephone you should:

a) _____

_____

b) _____

c) _____

_____

d) _____

_____

71. Incoming phone calls are the _____ of the salon.

72. It is important to answer the phone _____.

73. When booking appointments what information should you ask for?

_____

74. A practitioner is not available at the time a client requests. How can you handle this situation?

a) _____

b) _____

_____

c) _____

_____

75. When handling complaints over the phone, how should you respond?

_____

76. The tone of your voice must be _____ and _____.

BUILDING YOUR BUSINESS

77. What is advertising? _____

78. Advertising must _____

_____.

79. What is the best form of advertising? _____

80. What kind of advertising venues are available to salons?

a) _____

b) _____

c) _____

d) _____

e) _____

f) _____

_____

g) _____

_____

h) _____

i) _____

j) _____

k) _____

_____

_____

l) _____

m) _____

81. An important aspect of a salon's financial success revolves around the sale of

_____.